Acclaim f
Divine Mercy, Triumr

This refreshing book on Divine Mercy and cancer brings to life a truth so lacking today in the art of medicine — that addressing the spiritual needs of the sick and dying is paramount when we talk of healing. For the sick and their loved ones, this time of trial and suffering is one in which great trust in God is needed the most. Yet, for many, it is the time when they have it the least. This book is a must read for the sick, their families, caregivers, and especially those in the healing arts.

— **BRYAN THATCHER, MD**
Founder of Eucharistic Apostles of The Divine Mercy

What a wonderful combination: A knowledgeable physician and a faithful servant of God shares his insights on cancer and Divine Mercy. This book by Dr. Sobecks is a must have for all those who are dealing with a cancer diagnosis or great uncertainty. Being a healthcare professional and a cancer survivor, I realized our need to prepare in this life, so that we may be blessed with the gift of eternal life, as described in this book. I trusted in the love and guidance of God to help me through what was ahead of me.

— **KAREN ANN GLINSKI, BSN, RN**

This is a deeply moving book, written with grace, compassion, and hope. Dr. Sobecks has a true calling for the field of Oncology. It is clear to see that his life has been transformed as evidenced by compelling stories of interactions with his patients. As a fellow oncologist, I can attest that our patients and their families benefit immensely when one experiences the awesome power of prayer. Those who adopt the principles of this book will gain understanding and compassion. They will realize that God is in control.

— **JERALD KATCHER, MD**
Radiation Oncologist in Cleveland, Ohio

Divine Mercy, Triumph over Cancer could easily be subtitled *Triumph over Sin, Disease, and Trials*. It is an incredibly well thought-out treatise, not merely on death and dying, but on living. It is so comprehensive that it's like having a spiritual library of books all in one — complete sections on the Sacraments, growing in virtue, Divine Mercy, the Rosary, the 7 Sorrows, evangelization, and an appendix of prayers. A perfect book to buy for caregivers, family members, and those battling cancer or facing other difficult trials.

— VINNY FLYNN
Bestselling author of *7 Secrets of the Eucharist*
Director, MercySong Ministries of Healing

The God who created us is the God who redeemed us and heals us. Dr. Sobecks shows us how many ordinary people have found God's mercy amid the most difficult circumstances. We all want to be happy. We learn from these lives that our happiness does not depend upon our circumstances, but on our openness to God's grace, which is always available in abundance.

— MIKE AQUILINA
EWTN Host, Executive Vice-President, St. Paul Center for Biblical Theology

This dynamic approach to medicine by Dr. Ronald Sobecks incorporates Divine Mercy spirituality, the Sacraments, and medicine to offer meaningful insights on the treatment and spiritual care of cancer patients. Of special significance is the deep weaving of Sacred Scripture into patient care and specific examples of the healing power of the Sacraments. This is especially important to healthcare professionals who work long hours under difficult circumstances. They need to realize their work has a spiritual impact as well as meets the medical needs of their patients. This faith-filled book is a tremendous resource for healthcare professionals.

— MARIE F. ROMAGNANO, RN, BSN, CRC, CCM, CLCP
Founder, Healthcare Professionals for Divine Mercy

DIVINE MERCY
TRIUMPH
OVER
CANCER

This Book Belongs To:

Pancita
SeRapio

DIVINE MERCY
TRIUMPH
OVER
CANCER

A Guide for Patients, Survivors, and Their Caregivers

RONALD M. SOBECKS, MD

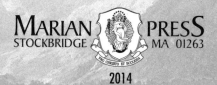

MARIAN PRESS
STOCKBRIDGE MA 01263

2014

Available from:
Marian Helpers Center
Stockbridge, MA 01263

Prayerline: 1-800-804-3823
Orderline: 1-800-462-7426
Website: www.marian.org

Imprimi Potest:
Very Rev. Daniel Cambra, MIC
Provincial Superior
The Blessed Virgin Mary, Mother of Mercy Province
February 11, 2011

Library of Congress Catalog Number: 2011924690
ISBN: 978-1-59614-237-4

Cover Design: Curtis Bohner
Cover Art: Composite rendering of Cuillin Mountains image ©2004 Ben Pfeiffer
and The Divine Mercy Image © Marian Fathers of the Immaculate
Conception of the B.V.M.
Inside Pages: Kathy Szpak

Copy Editing: Dan Valenti
Proofreading: David Came and Andrew Leeco

For texts from the English Edition of
Diary of St. Maria Faustina Kowalska

Nihil Obstat:
Lector Officialis
Most Rev. George H. Pearce, SNM

Imprimatur:
Most Rev. Joseph F. Maguire
Bishop of Springfield, Mass.
January 29, 1988

Printed in the United States of America

I dedicate this work to all patients with cancer
and to their families, friends, and loved ones
through the Divine Mercy of our Lord Jesus Christ
in the Most Blessed Sacrament and through
the intercession of the Blessed Virgin Mary.

Contents

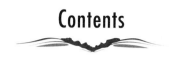

Acknowledgments

I am extremely grateful to Fr. Albert Tesek for all of his spiritual guidance and direction, which were of tremendous assistance as I prepared this work. In addition, I am forever thankful for the wonderful inspiration of my parents, Dr. Ronald and Mrs. Elaine Sobecks, as well as my wife, Nancy, and my son, Casey. I am also greatly appreciative to David Came, Dan Valenti, and the editorial staff at Marian Press for their insightful comments and suggestions. Finally, I am eternally thankful to Our Blessed Mother, the Immaculate Virgin Mary, and above all to Almighty God for His unfathomable Divine Mercy.

Preface

In the summer of 1992, during my fourth year of medical school at Case Western Reserve University, I made a visit to the tabernacle at Holy Rosary Church in Little Italy of Cleveland, Ohio. As I prayed in the church, an older woman I did not know came to me and gave me a copy of *The Divine Mercy Message and Devotion* booklet.

I didn't know it then, but this little action changed my life forever. From that booklet, I first came to know of our Lord Jesus Christ's message of mercy to the world through his faithful servant, Sr. Faustina Kowalska. I learned the Chaplet of The Divine Mercy as well as the importance of the daily Holy Sacrifice of the Mass and Eucharistic Adoration. I also came to understand the infinite value of prayer at 3 p.m., the Hour of Great Mercy, when our Lord Jesus expired on the cross. In addition, I became more fully aware of the value of offering sacrifices and sufferings for the reparation of sin. I was left in awe of the great mercy of God for all of us, particularly through the great Feast of Divine Mercy Sunday.

The Holy Spirit then guided me to pursue residency training in Internal Medicine in preparation for a career in Hematology/Oncology. Oncology is the field that focuses on cancer, while hematology encompasses diseases of the blood. Although as a physician I had expected to have the opportunity to help many patients, I did not realize how much the Lord God would teach me through these brothers and sisters of mine in need. The present work is meant to share with you a message of the sanctity of life and how Divine Mercy permeates all of our lives.

The Catholic Church teaches the importance of offering our sacrifices and sufferings in union with those of our Merciful Savior's during His Passion and death. As I have cared for many cancer patients, I have personally witnessed how many unknown saints there are in our world. These individuals live not for themselves but for others by bearing their crosses with patience and love, as Jesus did for us all.

Introduction

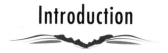

I often reflect upon how the Lord has increased my Catholic faith through the many people I have encountered in life. This particularly includes the many cancer patients and family members whom I have come to know as a physician. As I started my internship in Internal Medicine, my grandmother, Marian, was diagnosed with multiple myeloma (see Glossary).

This is a blood cancer that results in progressively lower blood counts and significant bone involvement that can be extremely painful. I had little experience with this disease at that time of my early medical training. However, I saw my grandmother gradually become frail as she wasted away from her disease. Although at times her bone pain was excruciating, she did not seek pain medications but tried to bear her suffering quietly.

I had known of her devotion to The Divine Mercy. As I reflect on her life, I am certain that her trust in this message from our Lord Jesus was what sustained her as she carried her cross. On one occasion, I spoke to a person caring for her, and with some humor, he wondered at times whether she was a "medical atheist" — one who didn't believe in doctors. My grandmother deeply believed God alone was her healer. However, gradually, she came to realize that the Lord uses those in the medical profession as instruments of His healing.

At the wedding feast of Cana, when Jesus performed His first public miracle, He could certainly have done it without the assistance of others. Instead, He used the servers to fill the jars with water. The headwaiter tasted it and declared it excellent wine (see Jn 2:1-10). Today, our Lord continues to use others as the means by which He makes His divine presence known, to impart His grace upon souls and bring about healing. My grandmother helped me to appreciate that the purpose of life is to know, love, and serve God so we may be with Him for all eternity.

I found it difficult to watch my grandmother, who was such a vibrant woman, become withdrawn as she approached her Good Friday. Nonetheless, in the midst of her trials, she was still open and giving. As I later pondered this attribute, I could not help but think of how her dying was similar to that of our Lord. I watched my grandmother refuse to take pain medication similar to how Jesus refused to take the wine drugged with myrrh as He was being nailed to the cross (see Mk 15:23). Just as Jesus had stretched out His arms and breathed His last, giving all He had for humankind, she also emptied herself and put her life into God's hands as she prepared to die. Despite her physical decline, an endless beauty radiated from her, for she like each of us was created in the divine image.

This experience of watching a loved one die from cancer helped instill in me a desire to pursue my career in Hematology/Oncology. The remarkable science and treatment advances in this field have inspired me, and working daily with many souls as they face tremendous challenges in their lives has confirmed my career decision. Cancer patients like my grandmother try to carry on with life each day despite having to bear their crosses.

That is the message of this book: the courage and strength that we receive from our merciful Lord to face our difficulties in life. I will return to this message repeatedly, and by sharing with you my medical encounters with people of tremendous faith and courage, I hope to leave you with a deeper appreciation for the greatness of Divine Mercy.

This book uses many references from the New American Bible, the *Catechism of the Catholic Church*, and St. Faustina's *Diary*. (Following the conventions of the *Diary*, the words of Jesus are in boldface, while the words of Mary are in italics.) In addition, I describe many of my personal experiences as a hematologist/oncologist with cancer patients, their families, and other healthcare providers. Only first names are used and in some cases pseudo names in order to maintain confidentiality.

Throughout the book, these personal examples as well as principles for cancer practice are juxtaposed with passages from

Sacred Scripture, Church teachings, and writings pertaining to Divine Mercy spirituality. This approach is intended to illustrate how the Gospel message and Divine Mercy should permeate every aspect of our lives as a common thread.

PART ONE

A Spiritual Approach to Dealing with Cancer

CHAPTER ONE

The True Means of Healing

Let me say it plainly: Those affected by cancer may triumph through Divine Mercy. These holy souls are often wonderful witnesses as to how one may live a life of and for Christ. Regardless of whether such patients are physically cured, their lives have great purpose in the divine plan of Almighty God. Furthermore, Divine Mercy is crucial for cancer patients and cancer survivors, and also for their families, friends, and healthcare providers.

Each of these individuals may face tremendous challenges from such illness. For some with cancer, there might be a drastic change in their former way of life. Uncertainty, anxiety, and various other mental, emotional, and physical sufferings may become evident. A number of them may experience frustration as they have to wait for treatment or become more dependent on others. Family members and friends of cancer patients are commonly affected as well. Things that they previously took for granted from their loved ones may no longer be possible due to their illnesses.

Healthcare providers likewise face many difficulties as they work with those who have cancer. These include interacting with patients and families from a wide variety of backgrounds. Each of them has his or her own unique social and cultural differences, often with distinct expectations and demands. In addition, these healthcare providers constantly require further rigorous training to remain current with science and technology in order to best care for their patients.

The Divine Mercy message is the definitive means for true healing. It strengthens and enlightens all who come to the Lord with trust. This wonderful message of mercy from God has always existed throughout history. Since the time of Adam and Eve's fall when sin first entered the world, humanity has continued to share in this original sin. Yet God in His infinite goodness and love willed that all may be saved and restored to Him through His mercy. As such, from the beginning, the Lord has continually revealed Himself to His people in order to let them know of His great love for them.

This revelation was made known through the prophets, the many holy men and women who have gone before us, and most clearly and perfectly in Jesus Christ. "And the Word became flesh and made His dwelling among us, and we saw His glory, the glory as of the Father's only Son, full of grace and truth" (Jn 1:14). Like many, I marvel at this reality. "For God so loved the world that He gave His only Son, so that everyone who believes in Him might not perish but might have eternal life" (Jn 3:16).

The Catholic Church has canonized some of the faithful who practiced heroic virtue and lived in fidelity to God's grace. These holy men and women serve as models and intercessors for all believers (see *Catechism of the Catholic Church*, 828). One such saint was Sister Maria Faustina Kowalska, who lived in Poland during the early 1900s and who was later canonized by Pope John Paul II on April 30, 2000 (Divine Mercy Sunday). Throughout the 1920s until her death in 1938, our Lord made known to her His great desire for devotion to His Divine Mercy, as well documented in the *Diary of St. Maria Faustina Kowalska*. Jesus entrusted St. Faustina with the mission to proclaim His message of Divine Mercy to the entire world as the last means by which He offers souls to avoid His just judgment.

Just as when thread is woven back and forth to make beautiful fabric, as we keep reflecting back and forth on the lives of those with cancer and then on spiritual matters, we can better appreciate how the two are directly related.

Since the whole person consists of both body and soul, it is necessary to understand that there is a balance between the two. If the soul of a person is sick from various sins (e.g., gluttony, sexual immorality, self-destructive practices including illicit drugs, etc.) this is reflected in the body, which often seeks after further evils of the flesh. This, in turn, may lead to further deterioration of the person's physical health. On the other hand, if the body experiences different ailments, this may have effects on the soul. The spirit is thus challenged to either give in to self-pity and despair or to rise to the occasion and offer up suffering for the love and glory of Almighty God.

I have constructed this book into four parts. The first presents a spiritual approach to dealing with cancer. How does one medically approach cancer? What are the general principles for its management? The book next compares sin to cancer, since both have the potential to destroy life. Just as it is critical to diagnose a cancer and characterize its type, so it is imperative that we recognize sin in our life to prevent it from causing the death of our souls.

Suffering is then contemplated along with freedom from imprisonment and the transformation of death into new life. Such hardships can be transformed by our Lord's great mercy and love for all humankind. We learn from Jesus that such suffering in the world is not to be considered a punishment from God. Rather, it represents an opportunity for us to demonstrate our true love for Him by offering it up for His greater glory.

Then, in part two, this book examines the means of spiritual help for those with cancer. Specifically, we consider how our Lord works through His holy Catholic Church in order to eliminate the chief ailment of the soul, which is sin. The power of prayer is contemplated as the means to unite oneself with God, who is the source of all life and healing. Particular attention is given to the Holy sacrifice of the Mass, the reception of the Sacraments, the intercession of Our Blessed Mother, as well as The Divine Mercy message and devotion.

Part three of the book reflects on how patients, their families, and healthcare providers may grow in virtue while struggling with cancer. This enables them to deepen their faith and better serve others as they offer what they themselves have received.

The final part of the book then focuses on how those affected by cancer may advance the kingdom of God. We see how after people experience Divine Mercy, they are called to be merciful to others.

At the end of the book, you will find a glossary of medical terms and selected prayers. The prayers are appropriate not only for those affected by cancer but for all as a source of healing.

The Catholic Church is the Body of Christ, which He Himself established. This divine institution should not be considered merely a set of buildings occupied by only an elect few, including the Pope, bishops, and priests. Rather, the Church is comprised of all believers from the past, present, and future who are united with our Lord Jesus Christ for all eternity. Therefore, when considering the Catholic Church, one actually identifies with all of its members throughout time and history.

This includes many souls from all walks of life such as a child with birth defects, an old widower who lives alone, a poor homeless woman who sits on the streets begging for assistance, and a sick patient suffering from cancer. For in each such individual dwells the holy presence of God, who gives great dignity and infinite value to the soul. Thus, each person must be deeply respected and loved as a child of God. Falling into sin not only weakens a person but the Church as well. Yet when a person does good, this further builds up the Church, which is the mystical Body of Christ (see Rom 12:4-5; 1 Cor 12:12-26; Eph 1:22-23; Eph 4:4).

Our Lord in His omnipotence knows well how best to heal, restore, build, and strengthen His sacred Body, the Church. This is accomplished by His infinite goodness, unfathomable Divine Mercy, and love for the world.

God created the world and judged it good (see Gen 1:31). The purpose of life is to serve Him and give Him the glory He so greatly deserves. As such, the Lord has used creation to make Himself evident to His children in the world. In particular, when Christ formed His Church, He gave her the Sacraments to allow souls to intimately encounter His divine presence throughout history. Jesus fulfilled the work of His Father by His death on the Holy Cross and then His Resurrection, which atoned for the sins of humanity.

This opened the gates of heaven for all who believe in Him. By restoring humanity to God from its fallen nature, Jesus allowed creation to be brought back to its proper order. Our Lord's Sacraments, therefore, use created matter as the medium through which He chose to reveal Himself to us. In Baptism, water, oil, and fire accomplish this purpose. In the Holy Eucharist, Jesus uses bread and wine. In Confirmation, Holy Orders, and the Anointing of the Sick, it is the sacred chrism that seals the recipient of the Sacrament. Of course, in all the Sacraments, the Lord uses various ministers. He created each of them as well to impart His grace through word and also commonly by the imposition of hands upon the recipients. The Holy Catholic Church has therefore always treasured and maintained the importance of the Sacraments. These are sacred gifts from our Lord that allow us to be restored and united with Him.

There are many types of cancers with many potential outcomes. These range from cure to temporary disease control to palliative care and hospice measures. Though different goals may be established for any individual patient, many with cancer find that at the time of diagnosis their perspective on life changes regardless of their religious beliefs. Our Savior Jesus Christ told St. Faustina to proclaim His mercy to the world. He told her that **Mankind will not have peace until it turns to the Fount of My Mercy** (*Diary*, 699). It is this message that brought my grandmother and so many others peace as they faced death from their cancers.

Furthermore, once we have experienced this great gift of Divine Mercy, we are to share it with others. Cancer patients and survivors, their families and friends, as well as healthcare providers may come to a new understanding of their purpose in life through this message of mercy. It is in showing mercy and living with compassion for others that Christ is made present to a world in such great need of healing.

Although many individuals may see similar people or things in the world, their encounters may be vastly different. One person may superficially glance at a particular event in life that another person experiences much more deeply. For instance, when one meets a person for the first time, the nature of the encounter may be merely one of salutation. However, for others, this may be an opportunity to get to know the person more intimately and then come to recognize the person of Christ Jesus in their midst.

I have been blessed as a hematologist/oncologist to know many courageous cancer patients and their families. Such experiences have opened my eyes to see the holiness of these individuals and have given me a heightened awareness of the sanctity of all life. The current work allows me to share a brief glimpse of the lives of many holy souls affected by cancer. Their courage and faith provide us with wonderful examples of how we are to trust in Jesus and His mercy in all circumstances and moments of life.

CHAPTER TWO

Coming Down with Cancer

Cancer is a condition characterized by the development of abnormal cells in part of a person's body. Other names for cancer that are routinely used in the medical community are malignancy, tumor, and neoplasia. Normally, healthy cells make up tissues, which, in turn, comprise different organs (e.g., the heart, brain, lungs, kidneys, skin, etc.) that make up the entire body. In each person, there is continual turnover with new cells being formed and old cells dying off. Thus, all things are maintained in a delicate balance known in medical terms as homeostasis. With cancer, however, this balance may be lost. Malignant cells may divide more readily than the normal cells that make up a particular organ.

In addition, these abnormal cells may be less likely to die and, therefore, they tend to have a growth advantage over their normal cellular counterparts. For instance, a tumor from colon cancer initially arises from transformation of normal cells that make up the colon. As these abnormal cells accumulate, they eventually form a mass. As the mass increases in size, it may affect other parts of the body nearby. This may result in pain, bowel obstruction, and perforation of the intestines, as well as bleeding that may be life-threatening. If the cancer is not fatal at this stage, it eventually spreads to other more distant parts of the body, such as the liver, lungs, bone, and brain. As the function of these other organs becomes impaired from the cancer, the patient's condition deteriorates and is ultimately fatal.

It is also important to understand that cancer is extremely diverse. No cancer is exactly the same. Malignancies that develop in each type of organ or tissue may behave differently from those that arise in other parts of the body. Some tend to grow slowly over months to years. These types often remain confined to a specific part of the body, as in the case of some cancers that develop in the skin or thyroid gland. Other malignancies may spread locally to nearby organs. Yet different types disseminate widely to distant parts of the body through the bloodstream and/or the lymphatic system. There are also diseases that are much more aggressive and grow rapidly. Some tend to form large tumors, while others travel quickly to various other parts of the body.

Cancer can also be broadly classified into two main groups. These include solid tumors and hematologic (blood) malignancies (see Glossary). The solid tumors are comprised of those diseases that .originate from solid organs. These would include cancers involving the breast, lung, intestines, prostate, bladder, kidney, ovaries, testes, head, neck, and others. The common hematologic cancers include leukemias, lymphomas, and multiple myeloma.

In general, solid tumors are considerably different than hematologic malignancies. They develop in a specific organ and with time gradually spread out of that organ. However, blood cancers such as leukemia arise in the bone marrow and then commonly exist in the blood. Therefore, at the time of diagnosis, these diseases are typically located throughout a patient's entire body.

Often as patients find themselves diagnosed with a cancer, they ask, "Why me or how did this happen?" For some patients, there is a well-known cause. This is certainly the case for those who develop lung cancer after having smoked cigarettes. In other cases, there may be a genetic predisposition to develop certain diseases such as for some types of breast and colon cancer. Individuals with family histories of these hereditary cancer syndromes are, therefore, recommended to undergo screening tests for these diseases (e.g., mammograms and colonoscopies) at much earlier ages than others.

Some tumors have also been associated with viral infections, as is the case for certain lymphomas that develop in patients infected with human immunodeficiency virus (HIV) that causes AIDS. Unfortunately, we do not know why many cancers develop or why they affect certain individuals. Much of cancer research is thus focused on improving our understanding of such diseases to subsequently develop new and more effective treatments.

When a person is diagnosed with cancer, it is natural for them to want to learn more about their condition. Patients may often seem overwhelmed at first, since they knew someone else who had cancer. Immediately, their minds may rush in many different directions. They commonly tend to expect that their lives will now become like the other person they knew who was affected by the disease. It is important, though, to inform them again that not all cancers are the same. In addition to letting them know whether their disease is aggressive or indolent, it is also necessary to instruct them that many other factors may influence how they will do with their cancer.

For instance, older patients may have a more difficult time with their disease than someone who is younger. On the other hand, age alone is not always predictive of poor survival for all diseases. Some older individuals, for instance, are otherwise healthy, and their cancers may be detected in earlier stages when treatment may be more successful. In fact, they may be much stronger physically, mentally, and emotionally than many younger patients. This may, therefore, allow some of them to tolerate treatment better. Moreover, a number of older patients may be more disciplined than others who are younger. Perhaps this may also enable some of them to be more compliant with following their doctors' recommendations.

Furthermore, patients with the same type of cancer may have different outcomes due to a variety of other factors. These include other medical conditions that affect their health, vastly different performance statuses, distinct genetic variations between their diseases, and differences in each patient's psychological background. By considering these few factors, one can begin to understand the great complexity that exists, which makes treating cancer patients extremely challenging.

In addition, when assessing the outcomes of a clinical trial with a new cancer therapy, it is important to recognize that the results may only pertain to the specific type of patients tested. For example, a drug may show efficacy in young men with a specific genetic subtype of leukemia who have a good performance status. However, this does not mean that the same treatment would be equally effective for elderly women with a poor performance status and a different genetic subtype of the disease.

For many cancers, the prognosis for a patient is directly related to their stage of disease. This also reflects how advanced their condition is at the time of diagnosis. There are different staging systems used in oncology for each type of cancer. Commonly, for many solid tumors, the stages are from 1 to 4. Stage 1 is typically localized disease, while stage 4 is widely disseminated throughout the person's body (also known as metastatic). For many malignancies, the more localized the disease is the better the chance that it can be treated and possibly cured. Even if incurable, diseases that are detected at an early stage may indicate that a patient would typically survive considerably longer than another patient with a more advanced stage disease. In addition, slow-growing cancers that are detected early may sometimes be observed without any treatment. This may potentially be for months or years, depending on the patient's clinical condition. In contrast, when there is widespread disease at the time of diagnosis, therapy is often indicated promptly.

There are many different therapies that are used to treat cancer. These include surgery, radiation therapy, chemotherapy, biologic therapies (see Glossary), and targeted therapies that have been designed specifically to interfere with a cancer cell's ability to survive. Sometimes different therapeutic approaches are combined, depending on the type and stage of cancer. Clinical trials are also commonly offered to patients, particularly if their diseases are incurable or without effective treatments. Since patients are the center of the team, it is important that they have a good understanding of their cancers as well as the best-recommended course of action to manage their disease.

CHAPTER THREE

Sin as a Type of Cancer

Many cancer patients go through periods of denial, thinking that nothing is wrong with them and that they do not have cancer. Similarly, many other people also deny that sin affects their lives. In either circumstance, whether a person does not seek medical help or spiritual help, there is gradual weakening of one's being that is ultimately deadly.

However, some patients with certain types of cancers, who are determined to fight their diseases, can be cured. Many of the treatments are difficult to undergo. For some, there may be significant risks of suffering and death. Often patients and their families struggle with much uncertainty as to whether they even wish to pursue these aggressive treatment options. If left untreated, most of these patients will die from their cancers.

Likewise, we all must decide whether we are willing to repent of sin in our lives. This is often difficult in that we have to change our entire outlook on life and make sacrifices. If steadfast in our approach, though, we can be successful in overcoming evil. Yet it is not us but Almighty God who heals us. Throughout history, the Lord has granted healing mercy to all sinners who turn to Him. For example, from Sacred Scripture, we see how the Lord manifested His steadfast love to the ancient Israelites.

This deep love that they experienced was known as *hesed*, based on God's faithfulness and goodness. God rescued them from their slavery in Egypt and brought them to the Promised Land. Over time, as they fell away, God did not abandon them. In His great mercy, He kept calling Israel back to Him through His holy prophets.

One must have a clear understanding of sin in order to be able to repent and return to the Lord: "Sin is an offense against reason, truth, and right conscience; it is failure in genuine love for God and neighbor caused by a perverse attachment to certain goods. It wounds the nature of man and injures human solidarity. It has been defined as 'an utterance, a deed, or a desire contrary to the eternal law'" (*Catechism*, 1849).

Furthermore, "Sin is an offense against God. ... Sin sets itself against God's love for us and turns our hearts away from it. Like the first sin, it is disobedience, a revolt against God through the will to become 'like gods,' knowing and determining good and evil. Sin is thus 'love of oneself even to contempt of God'" (*Catechism*, 1850).

Sin may be thought of as a spiritual cancer. Just as a malignancy left untreated may spread throughout one's body, so, too, sin can permeate an individual's being if there is no repentance. For instance, some patients with tumors involving the chest are at risk of death from their disease extending into and affecting the heart. Pride and selfishness are sins that may also start in one area of our lives and, if left unchecked, have free reign to destroy our hearts and cause spiritual death.

If sin can be thought of as a type of cancer, then it is naturally something to be shunned. The soul needs to recognize sin not merely as an imperfection but as a deliberate rejection of Almighty God. This realization should result in a holy fear of the Lord, which causes one to quickly repent from sin. Some patients who are ill may lose self-esteem when they find themselves disheveled or smelling badly. Yet these outward appearances are not important. Instead, it is the state of a soul that matters, for this alone will determine one's eternal destiny.

Those who seek purity and virtue properly prepare them-selves for everlasting life. Those who prefer sin, with no desire to repent and be reconciled with God, freely choose eternal punishment in hell. However, by accepting our states of life with humble obedience to the holy will of God and trust in His mercy, we may glorify the Lord greatly and atone for sin.

Saint Paul reminds us that we are all the members of the

Body of Christ (see Rom 12:4-5; 1 Cor 12:12-26; Eph 1:22-23; 4:4). As such, what one person does affects all the others. Those who do good help build the Body of Christ, while those who do evil weaken the rest. The issue becomes complex in that each of us is capable of doing good and bad, and we often do both. Though we cannot always change others, we can work to alter what needs to be changed in our own lives.

Those members of the Body of Christ who truly understand this often make great sacrifices to grow in holiness for the good of the entire Church. With each act of love and reparation, regardless of how small, healing and restoration to grace comes to others as well. Therefore, those who live devout lives may have a tremendous impact on others from their acts of love and mortification.

One may live in such holiness or alternatively in grave sin. However, God in His infinite love keeps calling each of us back when we stray from His care. The ultimate sign of God's mercy was His incarnation, when He humbled Himself to become man in the person of Jesus Christ. He proclaimed the message of His great mercy and love from His heavenly Father. Then Christ suffered, died a shameful death on the cross, and rose from the dead. Jesus has, thus, become the source of salvation for all who come to Him with humble trust. The Gospel message has proclaimed this eternal truth to the world throughout the ages. At the heart of this message are Divine Mercy and the Lord's infinite love for all. Many holy men and women have been wonderful witnesses of this reality, especially the Apostles, the Doctors of the Church, and the many saints.

One such individual was St. Maria Faustina Kowalska. She was a woman who came from a large family in Poland during the early 1900s. From a young age, she was called to pursue the religious life, and she later entered the Congregation of the Sisters of Our Lady of Mercy. Through the 1920s until her death in 1938, she received many revelations from the Lord regarding Divine Mercy as the last hope for the world. She recorded these in the *Diary of Saint Maria*

Faustina Kowalska. Although this great message of hope is not new, the Lord's revelations to St. Faustina were intended to increase the world's awareness of this tremendous gift in order for all of us to turn our hearts back to Him now. We then may receive healing and restoration to new life as we are freed from the bondage of sin.

Although St. Faustina lived a simple life, she is a marvelous example of one who loved God above all things. Her life was one of great trust in the Lord's mercy, and she teaches us how to develop a deep, personal relationship with Christ.

Father George Kosicki, CSB, summarized our Lord Jesus Christ's instructions to St. Faustina as the ABCs of mercy: **A**sk for God's mercy, **B**e merciful, and have **C**omplete trust in His unfathomable mercy. When people refuse to repent and trust in God's mercy, their sin is left "untreated." Since such souls will not let our Divine Physician heal them, they ultimately face eternal death. Cancer patients are often confronted with uncertainties regarding whether their diseases may be cured. However, when those who have lived in sin repent, trusting in the Divine Mercy and goodness of Almighty God, they can be certain that they will receive complete healing and forgiveness from the Lord.

The encouragement and support of others make it possible for cancer patients to pursue and complete difficult medical treatments. Likewise, prayers and spiritual direction from others such as priests, religious, and the lay faithful allow people to recognize sin in their lives and to seek God's mercy.

When I speak with patients who have acute leukemia, I often tell them that the bone marrow can be likened to a garden. The earliest stage bone marrow cells are like seeds that are planted in the ground. As the seeds grow and ultimately produce mature fruits or vegetables, so, too, the earliest cells in the bone marrow develop into fully mature blood cells necessary for life. However, weeds may infiltrate a garden, replace the area, and prevent fruit from being produced. In a similar manner, leukemia replaces the bone marrow space and eventually prevents normal blood cells from developing. Sin acts like this as well, as our Lord reminds us with His parable of the weeds sprouting up in a field of wheat (see Mt 13:24-30).

Leukemia cells are characterized by a lack of maturation and an inability to develop into healthy blood cells. Yet these cancer cells proliferate readily and, therefore, often fill up the bone marrow space faster than the normal blood cells can be produced. As such, the lack of red blood cell production results in severe anemia. This may cause patients to experience fatigue, shortness of breath, lightheadedness, and eventually heart failure. In addition, significantly low platelet counts also develop, which result in bleeding and easy bruising. As the number of healthy white blood cells becomes low, it leads to severe infections. Thus, leukemia that is not treated or that is not responding to treatment usually is fatal from bleeding or infection from progressively worsening bone marrow failure.

Similarly, sin often results from immature actions that are not remedied due to a lack of repentance and reparation. With time, even small sins that are not atoned for may be repeated. As these sins rapidly increase or proliferate in one's life, they, too, may eliminate any good that one possesses, which leads to death.

We recall in the Book of Leviticus (chapter 13) how those who had various skin lesions were often considered to have leprosy and, therefore, called unclean. These individuals were cut off from the normal Jewish life and in particular from entering the Temple, the center of their religion and their lives. Patients with cancer may also feel ostracized due to their illness. At times, they may perceive themselves as being "unclean" in the eyes of others and, therefore, removed in some sense from normal life around them.

Thomas was a patient under my care. He had kidney cancer that spread to distant parts of his body. In particular, the disease eventually involved his skin, and it manifested itself as large, black tumors. Thomas's wife remained close to him during the time of his treatments, and she had no fear of touching his wounds with her bare hands.

Many other patients have not only cancers affecting their skin but also various rashes and ulcers. Although cancer is not considered contagious like leprosy, often people still fear approaching those with malignant diseases. In former times, no one would touch a leper for fear of contracting the illness or becoming unclean themselves. However, this did not prevent our Lord Jesus from touching those with the disease in order to cure them (see Mt 8:1-4). Similarly, many family members, friends, and those who minister to the needs of patients do not worry about "catching" a cancer from the patients they touch. Rather, their focus is on caring for the sick with compassion.

This beautiful expression of love reflects the Lord's mercy alive and at work in our world. Just as sin behaves much like a cancer, it often also leaves sinners feeling like those with leprosy. For evil destroys the "spiritual flesh" of the one affected, and with time, it cripples the person further. This leads to separation from others and death. Only the Lord's mercy can free one from such disease.

When evaluating patients with tumors, advanced imaging studies such as an MRI or a CT scan can provide an accurate assessment of the location and the amount of disease that is present. As cancer therapies are administered, follow-up imaging studies can determine if patients are responding to their treatments. Carrie was a young woman I treated with Hodgkin's lymphoma. She had multiple enlarged lymph nodes. After she had received chemotherapy and a bone marrow transplant, her follow-up CT scans showed that the previously enlarged lymph nodes had disappeared.

However, years later, Carrie's disease recurred, and she was then successfully treated with additional therapy. This pattern of recurrent disease sadly is a common problem for many cancer patients. The initial therapy for some cancers may eradicate the vast majority of disease, but the small portion of disease that remains is resistant to that particular therapy. With time, the disease eventually grows back, and the next state of the cancer is worse than the first. With some malignancies, there are many different yet effective therapies available. Yet with each successive course of treatment, if the disease is not cured, it usually becomes more and more resistant until it is ultimately fatal.

In our spiritual lives, often our sins and shortcomings may not be obvious to us. As we find ourselves struggling, though, we eventually search for help. Jesus, our Divine Physician, often employs others such as family members, friends, priests, or religious to help us diagnose the problem. In many circumstances, one "test" may be insufficient to get to the heart of our problem. It may take multiple assessments by different individuals who "specialize" in various areas until we truly come to the root of our troubles and sins. Once detected, appropriate "treatment" must be administered. This consists of a thorough examination of conscience, repentance, an act of contrition, a good confession, and acts of reparation.

We must remain steadfast in our commitment to the Gospel of Jesus, or the cancer of sin will often resurface. For Jesus said, "When an unclean spirit goes out of someone, it roams through arid regions searching for rest but, finding none, it says, 'I shall return to my home from which I came.' But upon returning, it finds it swept clean and put in order. Then it goes and brings back seven other spirits more wicked than itself who move in and dwell there, and the last condition of that person is worse than the first" (Lk 11:24-26).

In order for successful outcomes in oncology to occur, patients need to be compliant with prescribed treatments. If patients do not follow their physicians' recommendations, they may jeopardize their chance of achieving a disease response or cure. When people ignore the Gospel message, they are also placing their spiritual lives at great risk. It is often striking to see patients meticulously follow instructions from their physicians to the smallest detail for things that are often of unproven benefit. Yet others place no trust in the commands of Jesus from the Gospel, which are of unquestionable, eternal benefit.

Another common problem that affects many patients with cancer is infection. For instance, patients with various blood cancers often develop low white blood cell counts that predispose them to what are called opportunistic infections. These usually consist of microorganisms that reside in patients' bodies or that are present in the environment and to which people are routinely in contact. A normal or intact immune system prevents an individual from developing infection from these pathogens (see Glossary). However, when a patient's immune system is significantly compromised from progression of their disease or from the toxicity (see Glossary) of their treatments, certain bacteria, viruses, or fungi may rapidly grow and lead to life-threatening illnesses.

In addition, some patients can be exposed to infections such as tuberculosis earlier in their lives. Although such exposures may not have resulted in active infections at the time, these patients may carry tuberculosis in their bodies for years or decades in a dormant state. Then, when their immune systems become compromised, some can develop active infections that may be highly contagious and rapidly fatal without prompt treatment.

Matthew was a man I cared for with a condition called myelodysplasia (see Glossary). This resulted in other repeated infections almost monthly due to his impaired immune status. As soon as he completed one course of antibiotics or antiviral therapy, he contracted another infection. Needless to say, Matthew spent much time in and out of the hospital for treatment. It often seemed he would never be healthy, which undoubtedly caused him great concern. Many with cancer share these uncertainties, particularly when they have lived with their diseases for long periods of time.

Similarly, for many individuals, sin and evil may repeatedly affect their lives. In particular, these souls may be attacked time and time again by temptations that weaken them spiritually. If a soul has a significantly compromised spiritual life, it does not have the capacity to withstand the many trials it will encounter. Just as cancer may be life threatening from the underlying disease, infection, bleeding, or toxicity from treatment, so, too, sin may be deadly to the spiritual life due to the devil's repeated insults.

Saint Faustina developed tuberculosis in the latter years of her life. This disease was a heavy cross to carry and eventually caused her death. Although tuberculosis is not a cancer, many of the sufferings that St. Faustina endured from this disease are similar to those experienced by cancer patients. For instance, in the 1930s, tuberculosis was incurable, much like many cancers. Saint Faustina experienced fevers, weight loss, fatigue, nausea, and intense pain. Furthermore, this disease isolated her from others. Perhaps even worse was the psychological stress she must have regularly endured, knowing that this disease would cause her death in the near future.

Those with cancer may, therefore, look to St. Faustina's example for inspiration. By invoking her aid, oncology patients may receive strength and better learn to imitate Christ as He embraced His cross.

Supportive care is often administered to cancer patients to help prevent infection or toxicity from treatment, giving these individuals a greater chance to overcome their diseases. Although many methods have been used to reduce the risk of infection, good hand washing remains among the most important. Failing to do this often allows the widespread transmission of bacteria from patient to patient, which may ultimately result in serious, life-threatening infections.

The effects of sin are similar. Without cleansing oneself from such evil through repentance and reception of the Sacrament of Reconciliation, a sin may rapidly spread throughout a person's being and result in spiritual death. In addition, the sin may be transmitted to others as easily as infection can spread from one person to another. Hence, there remains a critical need for good spiritual hygiene in order to maintain oneself in a state of grace.

Steadfast prayer, frequent participation at Holy Mass, the reception of the Sacraments, and other practices of Christian virtue strengthen souls. They then may withstand the temptations and storms in life that our Lord warned us of in the Gospel. Jesus told us that we must listen to His words and act upon them. In doing so, we may be like the wise man who built his house on a firm foundation of rock to protect it from rain, floods, and wind (see Mt 7:24-27).

When one's life becomes contaminated with sin, immediate repentance and reception of the Sacrament of Reconciliation are necessary. These are the means by which spiritual cleansing, renewal, and restoration to health are accomplished. The Lord's mercy is infinite and available to all. We must, therefore, seek it continually and help spread it throughout the world to help eradicate the epidemics and plagues of sin.

Although modern medicine has had many remarkable advances in the treatment of cancers, efforts to prevent such diseases before they even occur have been of paramount importance. Screening tests such as colonoscopies, mammograms, and PAP smears detect many conditions in either early stages of the disease or in pre-malignant states, when medical intervention may prevent or eradicate the cancer.

Similarly, we need to be in a "preventative" mindset when dealing with sin. By avoiding occasions of temptation, praying constantly, participating well in the celebration of Holy Mass, receiving the Sacraments regularly, and following the instruction of the Catholic Church and the Scriptures, we can prevent sin in our lives. The Lord told St. Faustina, **Most dear to Me is the soul that strongly believes in My goodness and has complete trust in Me. I heap My confidence upon it and give it all it asks** (*Diary*, 453).

As one focuses on cancer patients, we are not to stigmatize or label them according to their diseases, for in doing so one would neglect their dignity as human beings. We, therefore, continue to love the patient but hate the cancer by working constantly to eradicate their disease and restore them to health. In a similar manner, this has been how the holy Catholic Church approaches sin. We are to always love the sinner but reject the sin. All efforts should then be focused on a person's complete healing from the cancer of sin through our Lord Jesus Christ.

CHAPTER FOUR

Suffering

As I began medical school, I met and came to know a remarkable woman named Pat. Unlike many other students (including me) who began our medical education straight out of college, Pat had previously worked as a nurse for many years. However, over time, she was determined to change careers in healthcare and become a physician. This presented Pat with numerous challenges that included moving to a new city, giving up her prior source of income, and embarking on years of intense study. Furthermore, during medical school, Pat had to face many humbling circumstances. In particular, she often had to serve under numerous younger individuals who were medical residents or other healthcare providers with far less experience than her.

Despite these trials, Pat persevered with tremendous resolve and determination. I greatly admired her calm demeanor amid the daily turmoil and uncertainties that she encountered. I soon learned she had a strong faith in God that was central to her life.

After graduating from medical school, I also had the privilege to perform my Internal Medicine internship and residency training with Pat. As our medical careers advanced, we learned to care for many patients with various illnesses. Over the three years that we trained together, there were many sleepless nights while we were on call in the hospital. Although Pat was considerably older than me, in her late 40s, she endured well through these difficult times. She told me one day how much she would have liked to specialize in Hematology and Oncology. However, given her age, she decided not to pursue three more years of specialty training. Instead, she took a position in an

Internal Medicine practice. Pat was a wonderful physician and utterly devoted to caring for others.

About one year later, Pat became ill and had to stop practicing medicine. She began to lose much weight and to experience considerable pain with marked fatigue. When I learned that she was not well, I called her. She told me she had an advanced cancer — melanoma, an aggressive skin cancer. Pat then told me that prior to entering medical school, she had initially been diagnosed with this cancer in one of her eyes. A specialist evaluated her rare condition.

Although her initial treatments appeared effective, Pat had been left blind in the involved eye. I then marveled how she had gone through all her medical training with only one eye. Not only did Pat have to face the many other challenges of medical education, but she also was left with the constant uncertainty as to whether her cancer would recur. Then, after completing years of intense training and helping numerous patients, she faced imminent death.

The Christian Meaning of Suffering

One may ask, "Why?" Why should a person like Pat or anyone else have to suffer? What is the purpose of such painful experiences? One of the undeniable aspects of cancer is that with it will come suffering. This may include physical pain, emotional hurt, spiritual questioning, or the distress of loved ones witnessing a person's suffering.

Why do we suffer? People throughout history have pondered this question. It would seem, at least superficially, that nothing good could possibly be associated with pain and affliction. For the Israelites in the Old Testament as well as for many people in other cultures, such tribulations were commonly considered to be a reflection of evil or a form of punishment. If individuals found themselves having to endure turmoil or conflict, they could not have peace. As such, it only seemed natural that these events could not be good.

Pope John Paul II examined the Christian meaning of human suffering in his Apostolic Letter titled *Salvific Suffering*

(*Salvifici Doloris*, Feb. 11, 1984). From these reflections, one can come to an understanding that much good may emerge from suffering. Suffering, the Pope teaches, can be endured and accepted if it has meaning. Therefore, if the purpose of such hardship is understood, people may more easily be able to embrace and carry their crosses in life.

Those who study and work hard to earn a diploma or to achieve a good position at work frequently offer up many things to achieve their goal. Although at times their sacrifices may be difficult, as they remain focused on their goal, this suffering may seem like nothing. Saint Paul wrote, "The Spirit itself bears witness with our spirit that we are children of God, and if children, then heirs, heirs of God and joint heirs with Christ, if only we suffer with Him so that we may also be glorified with Him. I consider that the sufferings of this present time are as nothing compared with the glory to be revealed for us" (Rom 8:16-18).

Those with cancer or other life-threatening ailments may likewise embrace their crosses with true love. In doing so, their hardships may also seem like nothing when they consider their ultimate goal, life in Jesus. In contrast, if one constantly complains and vehemently resists such suffering without any love, their pain and anxiety are often intensified without bearing fruit. Jesus told St. Faustina, **It is not for the success of a work, but for the suffering that I give reward** (*Diary*, 90).

It is important to first consider how suffering came upon humankind by recalling the fall of our first parents, Adam and Eve. In the Garden of Eden, they had everything they needed. God had richly provided them with a beautiful place to live in His peace. Yet they fell as they were tempted by the devil to eat of the forbidden fruit from the tree of knowledge of good and evil. Rather than calling upon God for help and trusting in Him, they remained silent and obeyed the serpent, a creature, instead of God their Creator.

This pattern of fear and lack of trust was subsequently repeated throughout history by humankind. Despite Adam and Eve's fall, God did not abandon them. Instead, they were given the promise of one who would make things right again with God. The Lord told them that there would be enmity between the woman's offspring and that of the serpent. "He will strike at your head, while you strike at his heel" (Gen 3:15).

It has been said that this striking at man's heel is certainly a form of suffering. Thus, from the beginning, God gave us His remedy to atone for sin, and suffering was the means by which this would be accomplished as exemplified in the life of Christ. After Jesus' Resurrection from the dead, He walked with two disciples on the road to Emmaus. In their disappointment, they stated that they were hoping Jesus would have been the one to redeem Israel. The Lord then asked them, "Was it not necessary that the Messiah should suffer these things and enter into His glory?" (see Lk 24:21, 26).

As one reflects further on any sin, we understand it to be a turning away from God. The Lord is the source of all life, goodness, and happiness. By rejecting God, one also rejects all the good He intends to share with us. This is a grave mistake and an obvious cause of suffering.

In *Salvific Suffering*, Pope John Paul II states, "Man suffers on account of evil, which is a certain lack, limitation or distortion of good. We would say that man suffers because of a good in which he does not share, from which in a certain sense he is cut off, or of which he has deprived himself. He particularly suffers when he ought — in the normal order of things — to have a share in this good and does not have it. Thus, in the Christian view, the reality of suffering is explained through evil, which always, in some way, refers to a good."

Jesus said, "For God so loved the world that He gave His only Son, so that everyone who believes in Him might not perish but might have eternal life" (Jn 3:16). Pope John Paul II noted this "... refers to suffering in its fundamental and definitive meaning. God gives His only-begotten Son so that man 'should not perish,' and the meaning of these words 'should not perish' is precisely specified by the words that follow: 'but have eternal life.' Man 'perishes' when he loses 'eternal life.' The opposite of salvation is not, therefore, only temporal suffering, any kind of suffering, but the definitive suffering: the loss of eternal life, being rejected by God, damnation. The only-begotten Son was given to humanity primarily to protect man against this definitive evil and against definitive suffering. In His salvific mission, the Son must therefore strike evil at its transcendental roots from which it develops in human history. These transcendental roots of evil are grounded in sin and death: for they are at the basis of the loss of eternal life. The mission of the only-begotten Son consists in conquering sin and death. He conquers sin by His obedience onto death, and He overcomes death by His Resurrection" (*Salvific Suffering*, 4).

Pope John Paul II also distinguished human suffering into two general categories, physical suffering and moral suffering. In the case of physical suffering, the body of an individual hurts in some way. This may include things like headaches, chest pain, shortness of breath, fatigue, and all other ailments that affect the physical body. In contrast, moral suffering reflects pain of the soul. This may be experienced when one is depressed, anxious, undergoing psychological stress, or experiencing spiritual turmoil. Some encounter moral suffering through the various concerns of daily life or from the mental anguish of being misunderstood or not being accepted by others.

We also hear that suffering should not be considered as just something God uses for punishment. Pope John Paul II noted that in the Old Testament, Job had been innocent, but he suffered tremendously (see *Salvific Suffering*, 3). During his afflictions, he remained righteous and hence he gave glory to God, for which he was richly blessed. We also recognize that the Virgin Mary, who was without sin, underwent immense agony despite her purity. Her intimate union with Jesus enabled her to be united with Him in all things, including His suffering.

Jesus gave us the beautiful image of Himself as the Good Shepherd (see Jn 10:1-18). He stated that He will lay down His life for the sheep. No one takes it from Him. He said that

He has the power to lay it down and the power to take it up again. In these words, we come to more clearly understand that Jesus willingly accepted suffering for His Church. As members of His Body, we, too, are charged with accepting our own sufferings and crosses if we are truly to be His disciples.

Saint Paul wrote, "Now I rejoice in my sufferings for your sake, and in my flesh I am filling up what is lacking in the afflictions of Christ on behalf of His body, which is the church ... " (Col 1:24). One may ask what could possibly be lacking in the afflictions of Christ. After all, the Church believes that Jesus' perfect sacrifice of Himself through His Passion, death, and Resurrection is the source of salvation for all. However, we must also remember that as members of the Body of Christ, we have an intimate union with Jesus. This includes a share in His life, suffering, death, and Resurrection.

Pope John Paul II further elucidated this mystery: "In this Body, Christ wishes to be united with every individual, and in a special way He is united with those who suffer. The words quoted above from the Letter to the Colossians bear witness to the exceptional nature of this union. For, whoever suffers in union with Christ — just as the Apostle Paul bears his 'tribulations' in union with Christ — not only receives from Christ that strength already referred to but also 'completes' by his suffering 'what is lacking in Christ's afflictions.' This evangelical outlook especially highlights the truth concerning the creative character of suffering. The sufferings of Christ created the good of the world's redemption. This good in itself is inexhaustible and infinite. No man can add anything to it. But at the same time, in the mystery of the Church as His Body, Christ has in a sense opened His own redemptive suffering to all human suffering. As man becomes a sharer in Christ's sufferings — in any part of the world and at any time in history — to that extent he in his own way completes the suffering through which Christ accomplished the Redemption of the world.

"Does this mean that the Redemption achieved by Christ is not complete? No. It only means that the Redemption, accomplished through satisfactory love, remains always open to all love expressed in human suffering. In this dimension — the dimension of love — the Redemption which has already been completely accomplished is, in a certain sense, constantly being accomplished. Christ achieved the Redemption completely and to the very limits, but at the same time He did not bring it to a close. In this redemptive suffering, through which the Redemption of the world was accomplished, Christ opened Himself from the beginning to every human suffering and constantly does so. Yes, it seems to be part of the very essence of Christ's redemptive suffering that this suffering requires to be unceasingly completed" (*Salvific Suffering*, 5).

Therefore, Jesus' suffering and death were the perfect sacrifice for the salvation of all, which He accomplished once and for all. However, the Holy Spirit whom Christ gives to us continues to apply Jesus' work of salvation throughout history in His Body, the Church. Pope John Paul II stated that each of our sufferings, when offered up, is like a particle of Christ's suffering. This allows Jesus to continue His work of salvation through our lives.

Suffering in the Lives of Cancer Patients

Each of us can thus find any suffering that we encounter an opportunity to participate in the salvation of the world. We can either accept and embrace our crosses or try to run from them. Only the former choice allows us to conform our lives to that of Christ's life. God provides us with suffering as the means to rapidly advance in holiness.

Mark was a man who achieved a remission from his cancer. He and his family were delighted, and they knew that with more treatment he had the potential to be cured. However, Mark's cancer unexpectedly recurred, and he developed significant swelling in his right arm. This caused him significant discomfort, and he was hospitalized for further medical care. An ultrasound of his arm identified a large blood clot. Since this clot impeded the return of blood from the veins in Mark's arm, it had continued to swell. He then became short of breath, and further testing revealed that he had developed pulmonary emboli, which are blood clots in the lungs.

Many patients like Mark who have cancer may develop blood clots. The blood coagulation, or clotting, system is complex and normally maintained by a delicate balance. There are many components in this system that work together to maintain this balance that under normal circumstances prevents us from bleeding or clotting. These include platelets, the blood vessel surfaces, and various clotting factors. The clotting factors are proteins that come together when there is a cut or some other form of trauma that breaks blood vessels and results in bleeding.

This process can be likened to the formation of a large net. As platelets circulate, they can clump together in this "net" from the clotting factors to form a clot. This also attaches to the disrupted blood vessel area to prevent further bleeding.

Cancer is a well-known risk factor for the development of blood clots, and these may be fatal. Therefore, as in Mark's case, prompt medical treatment is imperative. Mark was immediately started on a medication called heparin to thin his blood. Although this therapy does not break down blood clots, it keeps the blood thin to prevent the clots from grow-ing in size or spreading. If the blood is adequately thinned, some patients' blood clots will completely resolve.

A concern for patients on blood thinners, though, is the potential to develop bleeding. For these medications interfere with the normal function of clotting factors, which may include their interactions with platelets. As such, while on this treatment it is as if only a loose "net" can be formed. This may be insufficient to catch and bind up circulating platelets to make an effective clot.

As Mark received further heparin, he began to bleed from a large catheter that had been placed in his chest for the management of his cancer. He then required a temporary cessation of his blood thinner and an infusion of plasma to replace clotting factors in order to stop the bleeding. Once this was accomplished and he was stabilized, Mark was able to receive further anticoagulant therapy at a lower dose. This allowed him to then continue treatment for his life-threatening blood clots.

Just as a delicate balance normally exists for the coagulation system to prevent excessive clotting or bleeding, our spiritual lives also need to be maintained in proper order. One who ignores or rejects any thoughts of a relationship with God is in grave danger of spiritual death. In contrast, those who focus only on spiritual concerns while neglecting others in the world who need them also fall short of the Lord who calls them to be merciful. Therefore, we must strive for this balance in our lives and trust in God, who helps us to achieve this end.

Mark not only endured tremendous physical suffering from his arm pain, swelling, shortness of breath, and bleeding but also considerable moral suffering. He was continually confronted with thoughts of his own mortality. Mark knew that his wife and family were distraught from his illness, and this undoubtedly contributed to his unease. Despite his physical afflictions and mental anguish, he maintained a positive attitude.

Mark was a man of great faith, and he let me know that this was the most important part of his life. He previously attended daily Mass and prayed regularly as he helped others to grow in their faith. With such faith and the intention of offering up his sufferings, he could carry on each day and further glorify Almighty God. Mark knew well that he was not alone during this time of trial. As he later faced death, he told me that he could not wait to see God face to face. His marvelous example of trust allowed him to participate in Christ's suffering and salvation of the world.

Jesus tells us that He is the vine and we are the branches (see Jn 15:1-10). Just as a branch cannot bear fruit when separated from the vine, neither can we bear fruit when separated from Jesus. We are told that the Father cuts away every branch that does not bear fruit, and the ones that do bear fruit He prunes so they bear more fruit. This should also help us understand why God allows suffering. The act of pruning dead or withered leaves and branches from a plant allows it to further flourish. However, this pruning is painful, particularly when it occurs in our lives. Yet through such suffering, God always brings about a greater good, which is the rich fruit of His kingdom.

How are we pruned? This may occur in many ways. Sometimes circumstances drastically change in a person's world. Perhaps this results from the loss of a job or failure in a project that we thought was important to accomplish. In other cases, this pruning may arise from a broken relationship. This may be with someone or a group of people who have been stifling our spiritual growth.

Sometimes our lives are further changed by the death of a loved one. This person who departed may have been a great source of grace for us, yet after their death, we may be able to move on to new horizons in life. Although one may have had a wonderful life together with their loved one who died, they are now given the opportunity to develop new relationships with others that may likewise be just as fruitful if not more so. The Lord may use such pruning to help each of us reach our full potential and help advance His kingdom on earth.

Sean was a man who experienced such pruning as he developed a highly aggressive lymphoma. This cancer involves the lymph nodes but may also spread to the bone marrow and other organs. Sean presented with a large mass in his neck, which horrified him. This may have caused his death rapidly if he had not been treated promptly.

He was transferred to our hospital, where he remained as an inpatient for one month. Initially, Sean underwent numerous tests and procedures. Although some of these caused him discomfort, the psychological effects of being pulled away from his normal life to face a life-threatening illness seemed far more devastating to him. Sean deeply missed his wife and two sons, whom he had to leave during this time.

As he underwent chemotherapy, Sean experienced nausea, vomiting, infections, hair loss, and fatigue. Yet at the end of the month, he began to recover. He then was found to be in a remission from his disease. After having a brief period of time at home with his family, he required more intense chemotherapy. With each treatment, Sean had more side effects. In particular, he developed a severe neuropathy (see Glossary), in which the nerves in his hands and feet were damaged. This caused him tremendous pain and limited his ability to walk and use his hands.

By the grace of God, Sean was cured of his cancer. He was able to return home to his family, and he was extremely grateful for all that the Lord had done for him. Sean, however, was left with his chronic neuropathy from which he continued to suffer. No medications or therapies were effective at eradicating his pain. He previously had been a mechanic, but he could no longer work to support his family. Despite the drastic change in Sean's life, he was a cancer survivor. He learned much from what he had suffered, and from such pruning, his faith life increased considerably.

The thought of suffering, however, is commonly regarded by many as something to fear and to avoid by all means. As we contemplate our Lord's Passion and death, though, we begin to realize the tremendous value of offering up hardships and tribulations for the glory of Almighty God.

Saint Paul helps us to understand this better: "For we who live are constantly being given up to death for the sake of Jesus, so that the life of Jesus may be manifested in our mortal flesh. So death is at work in us, but life in you. ... although our outer self is wasting away, our inner self is being renewed day by day. This momentary light affliction is producing for us an eternal weight of glory beyond all comparison, as we look not to what is seen but to what is unseen; for what is seen is transitory, but what is unseen is eternal" (2 Cor 4:11-12, 16-18).

Pope John Paul II also helps us to understand the other important aspect of human suffering in his Apostolic Letter *Salvific Suffering*. Not only do hardships and afflictions allow the one who suffers to have an opportunity to offer them up in union with Christ for the redemption of the world, but they also provide others the chance to show love and compassion to souls in need. Jesus clearly stresses the importance of having concern for others and offering them assistance in their need. He told us, "... whatever you did for one of these least brothers of Mine, you did for Me" (Mt 25:40). Likewise, in the parable of the Good Samaritan, Jesus illustrated how we should have sincere compassion for others (see Lk 10:29-37).

Pope John Paul II reflected on this parable in his apostolic letter as he wrote, "The parable of the Good Samaritan belongs to the Gospel of suffering. For it indicates what the relationship of each of us must be towards our suffering neighbor. We are not allowed to 'pass by on the other side' indifferently; we must 'stop' beside him. *Everyone who stops beside the suffering of another person*, whatever form it may take, is a Good Samaritan. This stopping does not mean curiosity but availability. It is like the opening of a certain interior disposition of the heart. ... We could say that suffering, which is present under so many different forms in our human world, is also present in order to unleash love in the human person, that unselfish gift of one's 'I' on behalf of other people, especially those who suffer. ... At one and the same time Christ has taught man *to do good by his suffering and to do good to those who suffer.* In this double aspect He has completely revealed the meaning of suffering" (*Salvific Suffering*, 7, emphasis in original).

Renee was a woman who had a relapsed blood cancer that later developed many life-threatening complications. While hospitalized, she had to have a bone marrow biopsy performed, which caused her great anxiety. As Renee under-went the procedure, a needle was placed into her posterior pelvic bone. During this time, her parents remained at her bedside, holding her hands and trying to reassure her that things would be fine. As the procedure was being performed, Renee experienced some discomfort.

However, her mother calmly kept telling her to offer it up. In particular, she told her daughter to think of the soldiers overseas constantly facing death, the victims of a recent hurricane, and little children with cancer undergoing similar tests. After these words of consolation, Renee seemed to experience a period of peace, which allowed her to tolerate the rest of the procedure without difficulty.

The importance of encouraging words during times of such affliction cannot be underestimated. We may consider how often in our own lives, we were able to endure a certain hardship or prevail over some difficulty merely from the words of someone the Lord sent into our life to offer us reassurance. This genuine concern for others amidst their trials in life allows one to bear Christ to the world.

Pope Benedict XVI has continued to help us understand the tremendous value of suffering. He stressed the need for trust in Jesus as he spoke to those who were ill at the Shrine of The Divine Mercy in Lagiewniki, Poland, on May 27, 2006. The Holy Father stated, "Dear friends who are sick, who are marked by suffering in body or soul, you are most closely united to the Cross of Christ, and at the same time, you are the most eloquent witnesses of God's mercy. Through you and through your suffering, He bows down to humanity with love. You who say in the silence: 'Jesus, I trust in You' teach us that there is no faith more profound, no hope more alive and no love more ardent than the faith, hope and love of a person who in the midst of suffering places himself securely in God's hands." (David Came, *Pope Benedict's Divine Mercy Mandate*, Marian Press, Stockbridge, Massachusetts, 2009, pp. 105-6).

Pope Benedict XVI then further illustrated the importance of suffering in his homily on Divine Mercy Sunday, April 15, 2007. He said, "The Lord took His wounds with Him to eternity. He is a wounded God; He let Himself be injured through His love for us. His wounds are a sign that He understands and allows Himself to be wounded out of love for us. These wounds of His: how tangible they are to us in the history of our time! Indeed, time and again, He allows Himself to be wounded for our sake. What certainty of His mercy, what consolation do His wounds mean for us! ... And what a duty they are for us, the duty to allow ourselves in turn to be wounded for Him!" (*Pope Benedict's Divine Mercy Mandate*, p. 38).

Later, Pope Benedict XVI also proclaimed how Jesus accompanies the sick during his homily at Lourdes, France, on

Sept. 15, 2008. As he spoke of the Sacrament of the Sick, he stated, "The grace of this sacrament consists in welcoming Christ the healer into ourselves. However, Christ is not a healer in the manner of the world. In order to heal us, He does not remain outside the suffering that is experienced; He eases it by coming to dwell within the one stricken by illness, to bear it and live it with him. Christ's presence comes to break the isolation which pain induces. Man no longer bears the burden alone: As a suffering member of Christ, he is conformed to Christ in His self-offering to the Father, and he participates, in Him, in the coming to birth of the new creation" (*Pope Benedict's Divine Mercy Mandate*, p. 108).

Love of others is the command that Jesus gave to us (see Jn 13:34). Such love is, therefore, how we are to approach all who are suffering, and it also remains at the heart of treating those with cancer.

Lessons from St. Faustina and Those with Cancer

Saint Faustina wrote in her *Diary*, "Oh, if only the suffering soul knew how it is loved by God, it would die of joy and excess of happiness! Some day, we will know the value of suffering, but then we will no longer be able to suffer. The present moment is ours" (963). She also wrote, "O my Jesus, I understand well that, just as illness is measured with a thermometer, and a high fever tells us of the seriousness of the illness, so also, in the spiritual life, suffering is the thermometer which measures the love of God in a soul" (*Diary*, 774).

Many cancer patients are familiar with suffering, and through its "school," these holy souls may obtain immense grace. Paula was a young mother of four children. She had undergone a bone marrow transplant for acute leukemia. Although she did fairly well for almost one-and-a-half years, she unexpectedly had a recurrence of her disease and abruptly faced death once again. In addition to her physical suffering, Paula was emotionally drained as well.

Yet this remarkable woman bore these hardships without complaining, and she maintained a deep sense of peace as she made plans to have her children cared for in her physical absence. Saint Paul tells us, "... the fruit of the Spirit is love, joy, peace, patience, kindness, generosity, faithfulness, gentleness, self-control" (Gal 5:22-23). Paula's long suffering gave her the opportunity to exercise great patience. This, in turn, allowed many of the other fruits of the Holy Spirit to become evident in her life. In particular, I marveled at her gentleness and self-control despite one worse turn developing after another in her life.

The last time that I saw Paula before she left the hospital and died, she hugged me and thanked me for everything. I initially felt somewhat perplexed, or perhaps even discouraged, since the treatment she had received failed to cure her leukemia. Later, as I pondered her words of gratitude, I realized she was comforted that she had not been alone during her difficult journey. Each small word of encouragement enabled Paula to carry her cross every day. By uniting her difficulties to those of Christ's sufferings and emptying herself of selfish concerns, her sacrifice was pleasing to our Lord.

The value of suffering cannot be underestimated. If we learn to suffer willingly for love of God and others, as our Lord requests of us, we transform what is seemingly evil or without purpose into a priceless treasure to be offered as a pleasing sacrifice to our God. Jesus' Passion and death on the cross may have seemed impossible to endure from the world's view. However, His true love for the Father and all humankind enabled Him to offer the perfect sacrifice of Himself for our salvation. We may offer our sufferings as a manifestation of true love, including love for our enemies and persecutors.

Saint Faustina wrote, "... [T]he purer our love becomes, the less there will be within us for the flames of suffering to feed upon, and the suffering will cease to be suffering for us; it will become a delight! ... for it is precisely when I suffer much that my joy is greater; and when I suffer less, my joy also is less. ... when we suffer much we have a great chance to show God that we love Him; but when we suffer little we have less occasion to show God our love; and when we do not suffer at all, our love is then neither great nor pure. By the grace of God, we can attain a point where suffering will become a delight to us, for love can work such things in pure souls" (*Diary*, 303).

Joan was a woman dying from recurrent leukemia. She showed patience and resolve as she offered up her sufferings. Although many others would have resisted such trials with great trepidation, her heart radiated with the joy of the living God. Each day, Joan seemed thankful just to have another chance to live for others. By offering them small words of reassurance or a simple smile, she would deeply touch their hearts. Her motivation appeared to be living the Gospel message in such a way that it brought others to Christ. Joan greatly loved her family.

Despite her need for more help as she grew weaker from her disease, she wished not to inconvenience them. She burned with love for others, and her selflessness helped transform those whom she encountered. Such souls quietly display the suffering face of our Lord Jesus Christ as He boldly underwent His Passion and death.

After the Lord warned St. Faustina to prepare herself for suffering, she thanked the Lord and replied to Him, "I am certainly not going to suffer more than You, my Savior. However, I took this to heart and kept strengthening myself through prayer and little sufferings so that I would be able to endure it when the greater ones come" (*Diary*, 488). By offering up mortifications, including various sacrifices and hardships throughout our lives, we may also gain endurance and fortitude. This, in turn, will help us to perform God's most holy will more perfectly.

Mary was a woman with cancer who exemplified one who was able to grow in such endurance from what she had suffered. She had developed toxicity from her chemotherapy known as hand-foot syndrome (see Glossary). Her hands turned intensely red and layers of skin began to peel off. This side effect was painful, and Mary was placed on an infusion of morphine. Although her hands improved with time, for a few weeks, she had limited use of them. As I spoke with Mary, she stated that she was thankful that only her hands were affected.

She then went on to tell me that when her son was just a child, he was severely burned over half of his body. He required a number of hospitalizations and skin grafting procedures during which time she remained at his side. Mary let me know that the discomfort from her hands, though painful, was nothing compared to what her son had endured. She and many other cancer patients thus demonstrate remarkable optimism in the midst of suffering, which is a wonderful example of courage and trust in the Lord's mercy.

On one occasion, our Lord told St. Faustina, **Those who are like Me in the pain and contempt they suffer will be like Me also in glory. And those who resemble Me less in pain and contempt will also bear less resemblance to Me in glory** (*Diary*, 446).

Fasting is an offering pleasing to God if performed with the proper intentions. Cancer patients often use fasting as a wonderful source of grace. Some patients cannot eat due to nausea and vomiting. Jim was one of my patients. He had a bowel tumor that resulted in an obstruction of his intestines. Like many others, Jim loved to eat. However, when trying to do so, he would immediately vomit.

Other patients like Jim may not be able to eat after receiving chemotherapy or radiation therapy due to significant toxicities of their mouths and intestines. For instance, many patients who receive high doses of such therapy prior to a bone marrow transplant may develop painful ulcerations throughout their mouths and throats. As such, they often require pain medications such as morphine infusions for weeks during which time they may take in nothing by mouth.

For some other individuals, there may be anorexia. With such a complete loss of interest in food, these cancer patients develop progressive weight loss and failure to thrive. This ultimately results in death. Still others may merely find food in the hospital unappealing and offer this up as a sacrifice.

Regardless of the reason for fasting, cancer patients may use this form of suffering to attain countless graces for themselves and others if offered with a true spirit of humility in union with the sufferings of our Lord Jesus Christ.

Numerous patients have given up many other things in life besides food as they faced their cancers. By reflecting on such individuals' lives, one can recall the words of St. Peter, "We have given up everything and followed You." Our Lord Jesus then replied, "Amen, I say to you, there is no one who has given up house or brothers or sisters or mother or father or children or lands for My sake and for the sake of the Gospel who will not receive a hundred times more now in this present age: houses and brothers and sisters and mothers and children and lands, with persecutions, and eternal life in the age to come. But many that are first will be last, and the last will be first" (Mk 10:28-31).

Saint Paul said of his own suffering, "... a thorn in the flesh was given to me, an angel of Satan, to beat me, to keep me from being too elated. Three times I begged the Lord about this, that it might leave me, but He said to me, 'My grace is sufficient for you, for power is made perfect in weakness.' I will rather boast most gladly of my weaknesses, in order that the power of Christ may dwell within me. Therefore, I am content with weaknesses, insults, hardships, persecutions, and constraints, for the sake of Christ; for when I am weak, then I am strong" (2 Cor 12:7-10).

Cancer patients may find great consolation in these words. They, too, may have multiple thorns in their flesh, including their diseases, the treatment that they face, the strained relationships that they must endure as well as the many uncertainties in their lives. However, they may also be confident that the grace of Christ Jesus will be more than adequate to enable them to endure all hardships and trials. For instance, many patients require being stuck repeatedly for blood draws or to have intravenous lines placed that may result in considerable discomfort. As such, they may reflect on our Lord Jesus who patiently endured the piercing of His sacred flesh with nails during His Crucifixion.

Paul was a man who I helped care for with an aggressive lymphoma that was life threatening. However, his family life at home was worse than this disease. He told me that he had a wife and a 6-year-old daughter whom he loved dearly. His wife was an alcoholic, though, and she had an extremely difficult time coping with his disease. In fact, she sought to divorce him right after he had been hospitalized for a month to undergo a bone marrow transplant. Although Paul may have been cured of his disease, he still had to endure further suffering.

Each day was filled with considerable anxiety for him. He continually asked himself why he was being rejected. Amidst these trials, Paul learned humility, and he displayed tremendous gratitude to those who had cared for him. He, like many other patients, felt that his disease was not only attacking him physically but was also threatening his inner being through its destruction of his family relationships and his identity as a person. Likewise, sin not only harms one part of our life. It also permeates through other dimensions of who we are as well. If left unchecked, it eventually may affect others, particularly those whom we love most.

Paul's family life was extremely challenging, with new concerns developing repeatedly. Though free from his cancer, he faced further inner turmoil. Paul constantly told me again and again that he loved his wife. However, her problems with alcohol abuse had not only contributed to their marital problems but were also affecting their young daughter. He strived to be a good example to his little girl amidst the pain of his impending divorce. Although at times, he may have felt that his efforts were futile, in fact, they had an effect. In addition to being a model for others who face affliction, I feel that Paul grew interiorly from this painful experience.

He could find support from the Sacred Scriptures by reflecting upon the words of wisdom and consolation that they provide. "Consider it all joy, my brothers, when you endure various trials, for you know that the testing of your faith produces perseverance. And let perseverance be perfect, so that you may be perfect and complete, lacking in nothing" (Jas 1:2-3).

Further, St. Paul tells us, "I consider that the sufferings of this present time are as nothing compared with the glory to be revealed for us. ... What will separate us from the love of Christ? Will anguish, or distress, or persecution, or famine, or nakedness, or peril, or the sword? As it is written, 'For Your sake we are being slain all the day; we are looked upon as sheep to be slaughtered.' No, in all these things we conquer overwhelmingly through Him who loved us. For I am convinced that neither death, nor life, nor angels, nor principalities, nor present things, nor future things, nor powers, nor height, nor depth, nor any other creature will be able to separate us from the love of God in Christ Jesus our Lord" (Rom 8:18, 35-39).

Many patients with cancer may become depressed. For some, this may require specific medication or counseling with a therapist or psychiatrist. However, such periods, which may be particularly trying, should not result in despair. For these times may be opportunities for immense spiritual growth.

Betty was a woman with an extremely vibrant personality. However, she repeatedly encountered disappointments and role losses over the years as she struggled with complications from her cancer treatment. Because of a prolonged hospitalization, Betty first missed her son's wedding. Later, she developed worsening weakness and difficulty breathing. This significantly limited her ability to perform her usual activities at home. With time, she required more and more assistance to simply care for herself.

Eventually, this necessitated that she leave her home in order to be cared for in a nursing facility. Betty's sparkling personality gradually became subdued. In fact, even though physically she had been stabilized and seemed to be doing well, she became withdrawn from others. Her family found this to be frustrating.

Despite her gradual decline, I could sense her strong faith in God. I tried to offer Betty some encouraging words, including further support for her to persist in her prayers. About a month later, when she had returned for a follow-up appointment to see me, she had been completely transformed. Her personality once again was filled with life, though nothing had changed with her physical condition. It seemed clear that her change of heart occurred as she persisted in prayer amidst her suffering.

Many great saints, including St. Faustina, encountered further struggles during what is called the dark night of the soul. In her *Diary*, St. Faustina wrote, "The heaviest suffering for me was that it seemed to me that neither my prayers nor my good works were pleasing to God. I did not dare lift up my eyes to heaven" (68). She also noted, "That priest consoled me, saying that in my present situation I was more pleasing to God than if I were filled with the greatest consolations. 'It is a very great grace, Sister,' he told me, 'that in your present condition, with all the torments of soul you are experiencing, you not only do not offend God, but you even try to practice virtues. I am looking into your soul, and I see God's great plans and special graces there; and seeing this, I give thanks to the Lord.' But despite all that, my soul was in a state of torture; and in the midst of unspeakable torments, I imitated the blind man who entrusts himself to his guide, holding his hand firmly, not giving up obedience for a single moment, and this was my only safety in this fiery trial" (*Diary*, 68).

She later wrote, "One thing did surprise me: it often happened that, at the time when I was suffering greatly, these terrible torments would disappear suddenly just as I was approaching the confessional; but as soon as I had left the confessional, all these torments would again seize me with even greater ferocity. I would then fall on my face before the Blessed Sacrament repeating these words: 'Even if You kill me, still will I trust in You!'" (*Diary*, 77).

She then noted, "'Do what You will with me, O Jesus, I will adore You in everything. May Your will be done in me, O my Lord and my God, and I will praise Your infinite mercy.' Through this act of submission, these terrible torments left me. Suddenly I saw Jesus, who said to me, **I am always in your heart.** An inconceivable joy entered my soul, and a great love for God set my heart aflame. I see that God never tries us beyond what we are able to suffer. Oh, I fear nothing; if God sends such great suffering to a soul. He upholds it with an even greater grace, although we are not aware of it. One act of trust at such moments gives greater glory to God than whole hours passed in prayer filled with consolations. Now I see that if God wants to keep a soul in darkness, no book, no confessor can bring it light" (*Diary*, 78).

Bill was a man I helped take care of who had a strong faith in God and a deep love of the Sacred Scriptures. He had been hospitalized for weeks to receive treatment for his cancer. During this time, I had spoken to Bill about moral suffering from which one may experience intense mental anguish. He then reminded me that Jesus, too, had to go out into the desert for 40 days before His public ministry began. During this time, He had been tempted by the devil (see Lk 4:1-13).

Each day, Bill faced new uncertainties while hospitalized. He wondered if he would ever go home. He asked if he could ever travel or simply do the things that he was accustomed to doing. At times, he was likely tempted to doubt. Yet he tried consistently to take one day at a time and face the challenges of each moment. He had a wonderful family and many friends who continually visited him to offer him support. Despite these blessings, Bill struggled as he tried to cope with his illness. However, he gained strength by reflecting on our Lord's tremendous resolve and perseverance as He Himself was tempted in the desert.

Patients struggling with cancer or with any other illness can also draw great consolation and strength from the words that our Lord spoke to St. Faustina during the time of her suffering. Jesus stated, **Poor soul, I see that you suffer much and that you do not have even the strength to converse with Me. So I will speak to you. Even though your sufferings were very great, do not lose heart or give in to despondency. But tell Me, My child, who has dared to wound your heart? Tell Me about everything, be sincere in dealing with Me, reveal all the wounds of your heart. I will heal them, and your suffering will become a source of your sanctification** (*Diary*, 1487).

Saint Faustina then said, "Lord, my sufferings are so great and numerous and have lasted so long that I have become discouraged."

Jesus, in turn, replied, **My child, do not be discouraged. I know your boundless trust in Me; I know you are aware of My goodness and mercy. Let us talk in detail about everything that weighs so heavily upon your heart.**

She then said, "There are so many different things that I do not know what to speak about first, nor how to express it."

Our Lord responded, **Talk to Me simply, as a friend to a friend. Tell Me now, My child, what hinders you from advancing in holiness?**

Saint Faustina then stated, "Poor health detains me on the way to holiness. I cannot fulfill my duties. I am as useless as an extra wheel on a wagon. I cannot mortify myself or fast to any extent, as the saints did. Furthermore, nobody believes I am sick, so that mental pain is added to those of the body, and I am often humiliated. Jesus, how can anyone become holy in such circumstances?" (*Diary*, 1487)

Jesus then told her, **True, My child, all that is painful. But there is no way to heaven except the way of the cross. I followed it first. You must learn that it is the shortest and surest way.**

She then stated, "Lord, there is another obstacle on the road to holiness. Because I am faithful to You, I am persecuted and suffer much."

Jesus responded, **It is because you are not of this world that the world hates you. First it persecuted Me. Persecution is a sign that you are following in My footsteps faithfully.**

She next said, "My Lord, I am also discouraged because neither my superiors nor my confessor understand my interior trials. A darkness clouds my mind. How can I advance? All this discourages me from striving for the heights of sanctity." (*Diary*, 1487)

The Lord then said, **Well, My child, this time you have told Me a good deal. I realize how painful it is not to be understood, and especially by those whom one loves and** with whom one has been very open. But suffice it to know that I understand all your troubles and misery. I am pleased by the deep faith you have, despite everything, in My representatives. Learn from this that no one will understand a soul entirely — that is beyond human ability. Therefore, I have remained on earth to comfort your aching heart and to fortify your soul, so that you will not falter on the way. You say that a dense darkness is obscuring your mind. But why, at such times, do you not come to Me, the light who can in an instant pour into your soul more understanding about holiness than can be found in any books? No confessor is capable of teaching and enlightening a soul in this way.

Know, too, that the darkness about which you complain I first endured in the Garden of Olives when My Soul was crushed in mortal anguish. I am giving you a share in those sufferings because of My special love for you and in view of the high degree of holiness I am intending for you in heaven. A suffering soul is closest to My Heart (*Diary*, 1487).

She then replied, "One more thing, Lord. What should I do when I am ignored and rejected by people, especially by those on whom I had a right to count in times of greatest need?" (*Diary*, 1487).

Jesus told her, **My child, make the resolution never to rely on people. Entrust yourself completely to My will saying, 'Not as I want, but according to Your will, O God, let it be done unto me.' These words, spoken from the depths of one's heart, can raise a soul to the summit of sanctity in a short time. In such a soul I delight. Such a soul gives Me glory. Such a soul fills heaven with the fragrance of her virtue. But understand that the strength by which you bear sufferings comes from frequent Communions. So approach this fountain of mercy often, to draw with the vessel of trust whatever you need** (*Diary*, 1487).

Saint Faustina then said, "Thank You, Lord, for Your goodness in remaining with us in this exile as the God of mercy and blessing us with the radiance of Your compassion and goodness. It is through the light of Your mercy that I have come to understand how much You love me" (*Diary*, 1487).

Patients with cancer may thus rejoice amidst their sufferings, which provide them the opportunity to be closely united with our Lord, the source of all love and mercy.

Some cancer patients use their time of illness as an opportunity to advance in holiness as they work continuously to increase their faith. Many of them may spend hours in prayer and contemplation, closing out the distractions of the world that previously had prevented them from receiving more graces and faith from the Lord God.

Mike was a man who had been hospitalized for many weeks in order to receive treatment for recurrent cancer. As each day passed, he would wonder how long he had to live. He also repeatedly asked whether he should undergo further treatment, given the potential risks of various side effects from such therapy. In addition, he had to decide was it even worth undergoing treatment if he could die from it and never leave the hospital. Of course, further chemotherapy would also require him to have numerous tests performed such as multiple blood draws in order to monitor his clinical condition. This, along with radiology tests and potential consultations from various other specialists, would add more and more inconveniences to his life.

All of these things weighed heavily on his mind and greatly contributed to his anxiety. However, during this time, Mike also read about St. Padre Pio. Mike tried to pray for the intercession of St. Padre Pio to assist him in his difficulties. Through the Communion of Saints, Mike could be united with St. Padre Pio. All of the faithful likewise share in this spiritual union, which exists due to God's great mercy and love.

Though the world seeks peace from wars and those in oncology fight to win the battle against cancer, spiritual warfare will continue to exist until God's kingdom finally comes in its fullness. Therefore, cancer patients like others must struggle daily not only against evil in the world but also against complacency and sin. Their efforts may be more fruitful as they follow the instruction given to St. Faustina. For she was told, "... do everything with the pure intention of reparation for poor sinners. This keeps me in continual union with God, and this intention perfects my actions, because everything I do is done for immortal souls. All hardships and fatigue are as nothing when I think that they reconcile sinful souls with God" (*Diary*, 619).

As Our Most Blessed Mother, Mary stayed at the foot of Jesus' cross. We, too, can stay at the feet of our suffering brothers' and sisters' crosses. We may not be able to truly appreciate how horrible Jesus' suffering on the cross must have been, but when we stay at the side of those suffering, we can experience our Lord's anguish. Just as His great mercy was poured out as blood and water from the cross onto the world (see *Diary*, 848), it also continues to gush forth from His Most Sacred Heart upon us through others. Hence, the Lord God can always bring a far greater good out of any evil.

Although the sufferings cancer patients endure may weaken them physically, their spiritual lives may be greatly enriched, and this will profit them for all eternity. As they offer up these trials to the Lord with hearts full of love, they imitate Jesus and are transformed into His likeness. This allows them then to bear Christ more and more to the world around them.

CHAPTER FIVE

Freedom from Imprisonment

Jerry was a man with an aggressive cancer who came to me for further evaluation. As we spoke during our first encounter, he informed me that many years prior to our meeting, he had used several types of recreational drugs. However, Jerry went on to tell me that he had later found Jesus Christ, and his life was completely transformed. He gave up his addictive substances and began to minister and evangelize in prisons. Although he may not have been physically incarcerated in a jail, his past addictions had restricted his freedom and in essence had imprisoned him. By reaching out to inmates in various prisons, Jerry brought the light of Christ into these abodes of darkness. Similarly, our Lord tells us that if we commit sin, we are slaves to sin (see Jn 8:34). A slave is confined against his or her will, often without any hope, but our Lord's mercy is our never-failing hope.

It is sad to think that those who are incarcerated are often completely abandoned by society, including those who are imprisoned for only minor offenses. Although these individuals need to complete their prison sentences for justice's sake, ideally, this period of confinement should provide an opportunity for repentance and spiritual renewal. Our Lord's mercy is readily available for these prisoners. Even if society is unable to forgive their offenses, the Lord's ways are not man's ways and the Lord's thoughts are not man's thoughts (see Is 55:8). Jesus welcomes these lost sheep and prodigal sons and daughters back into His fold as they repent and return to Him trusting in His mercy.

Some cancer patients may at times feel imprisoned as well. However, if they also turn to Jesus our Good Shepherd, they will find true freedom. As others come to visit them, their spirits may be refreshed. The corporal works of mercy from our Lord include visiting the sick and imprisoned, which may be accomplished through our works, words, and prayer. Unfortunately, sometimes we may have narrow viewpoints when we consider those who are imprisoned or physically infirm. Our prayers and sacrifices must also be offered up to help free us from the imprisonment that comes from stereotyping, complacency, and a lack of forgiveness.

We must recall that a number of the Church's greatest saints were prisoners at some time during their lives. Saint John the Baptist boldly proclaimed the truth, which resulted in his arrest by King Herod, who subsequently had him executed. Saints Peter, John, and other Apostles were also arrested for their witness to the risen Lord Jesus.

Saint Paul, who preached the Gospel message to the Gentiles, likewise was rewarded by the chains of imprisonment. He tells us, "Remember Jesus Christ, raised from the dead, a descendant of David: such is my gospel, for which I am suffering, even to the point of chains, like a criminal. But the word of God is not chained. Therefore, I bear with everything for the sake of those who are chosen, so that they too may obtain the salvation that is in Christ Jesus, together with eternal glory" (2 Tim 2:8-10).

Of course, most notable for His imprisonment was our Lord Jesus Christ. He accepted being arrested and brutally tortured during His period of confinement prior to His crucifixion. By offering up trials such as these, one may receive unimaginable graces.

Though St. Faustina was not imprisoned for any crime, we learn from her *Diary* that she commonly was confined to her room in the convent and later within infirmaries due to her tuberculosis. In these holy places, our Lord Jesus frequently communed with her despite the humble measure of those quarters. It was in her convent cell that she offered up terrible sufferings for the spiritual benefit of other souls. Saint Faustina may, therefore, serve as a role model for patients with other serious, life-threatening diseases. In such confined environments, one may avoid the distractions of the world and focus his or her life more clearly on our Lord God.

Some people are imprisoned by sin, doubt, fear, and other vices. Saint Faustina noted an elderly sister who had been suffering interiorly for years due to uncertainty as to whether God had forgiven her for her sins. She had doubted the words of her confessors who told her to be at peace. Due to this sister's persistence, St. Faustina promised her that she would pray for her. Our Lord replied to St. Faustina during Benediction, **Tell her that her disbelief wounds My Heart more than the sins she committed** (*Diary*, 628). So must we repent from our sins and then have complete trust in our Lord's mercy and infinite goodness if we are to be free from evil.

Imprisonment from one's passions and the things of the flesh allows for the virtue of humility to be perfected. This self-abasement may cultivate the good soil that Jesus referred to in His parable of the sower and the seed. When such souls hear the Word of God, they may then produce a rich yield of 30-, 60- and 100-fold as they help further the kingdom of Almighty God upon the earth (see Mk 4:1-20).

Matt was a young man who had a blood disorder called myelodysplasia (see Glossary). The disease resulted in profoundly low blood counts that significantly impaired his immune system. He developed recurrent serious infections, including a severe pneumonia. At times, this necessitated that he be isolated in a hospital room with respiratory precautions to help prevent him from spreading the infection to others. Before his cancer diagnosis, Matt had a hard life. He came from a home where his parents got divorced, and he became addicted to drugs and alcohol by age 16. During that time, he also had a child with his girlfriend. He like many others had relied on these various passions of the flesh as a means of coping in life.

Despite his rough beginning, Matt was gradually transformed spiritually by his disease. He learned to read the Word of God, and he began to wear a cross. As his healthcare providers grew to know him better, their relationships with him became much more positive. As we watched him suffer, our hearts melted. He, in turn, helped us to demonstrate compassion, concern, and love. Matt's prolonged hospital confinement helped me to better appreciate what St. Faustina's time of illness must have been like during the isolation to treat her tuberculosis. In solitude, her soul was transformed into that of a great saint, for she was not alone in her most difficult trials. Faustina, Matt, and anyone else who confidently trusts in the Lord are never alone.

Many patients with cancer may also feel locked up with concerns regarding their treatment. Often their therapies are extremely expensive and, unfortunately in most cases, samples of medications are not available. For others, there are no standard treatments for their diseases. As such, clinical trials are frequently offered that may not be covered by patients' medical insurance companies. In other cases, effective and potentially curative therapy such as a bone marrow transplant exists to treat some diseases. However, those without medical insurance coverage may not be able to receive such treatments. Although problems may exist with financial coverage for some patients' medical care, they may apply for Medicaid to receive support from the government.

These uncertainties may add to their anxiety when they are already dealing with significant stress from their cancers. However, our Lord's mercy and healing are free for all who approach this fount of graces with complete trust. No soul that seeks Him is "denied coverage" from His mercy and love. These unfathomable graces are continually being poured out on the world.

In particular, those souls who immerse themselves completely in Jesus' mercy, adoring it and glorifying it, are pleasing to the Lord for their obedience (see *Diary*, 1572). To have a deep confidence in the Lord is a true gift. For such souls who have no doubts in God's mercy do not live in fear, but rather in trust. They do not live as slaves but as children of God (see Rom 8:14-17).

Slavery may take many forms in life. In oncology, perhaps one of the most notable types is the addiction to cigarette smoking. This has been found to be the cause of multiple fatal cancers and many other life-threatening healthcare problems as well. John was a man who had been treated for head and neck cancer. He required the placement of a tracheostomy (see Glossary) after his cancer was diagnosed. This necessitated an incision being made in the front of his neck to make a hole through which an artificial airway could be placed in order for him to breathe. Despite not being able to speak normally after the procedure, John continued to smoke cigarettes through his tracheostomy due to his strong addiction. Many other cancer patients have shared this same self-destructive behavior, which resulted in premature death.

Those who live in a state of mortal sin likewise continue to indulge in further evil that ultimately results in spiritual death. However, just as those who smoke cigarettes may break the addiction with discipline and support from others, those who live in serious sin may be set free through sincere repentance, the reception of the Sacrament of Reconciliation, and complete trust in our Lord's mercy.

After Jesus called St. Matthew to abandon his former way of life as a tax collector and to follow Him, Jesus went to St. Matthew's home. There He ate with other tax collectors, which caused the Pharisees to ask why Jesus ate with sinners. Our Lord responded to them that the sick need a physician, not those who are well. Then Jesus told them, "Go and learn the meaning of the words, 'I desire mercy, not sacrifice'" (see Mt 9:9-13).

Ron was a man who I came to know in oncology. He eventually gained an understanding of these words of Jesus, "I desire mercy, not sacrifice." Ron was meticulous. He always tried to control things in life. He made extensive plans to structure his life and the world around him. This included the projects that he wanted to accomplish at work each day, the social events he desired to arrange, as well as the time he allotted for sharing his life with others.

In particular, Ron told me that his drive for structure in the world around him often caused friction with others. He specifically noticed this at home, when he found that his family did not always conform to his expectations. Although his intentions may often have been good, Ron had to learn the importance of not always getting his way.

As he reflected on his life, it became apparent that he often felt imprisoned by his fear and lack of control of many things. Ron let me know that he had a deep spiritual life, and he greatly treasured his Catholic faith. Despite these treasures, he still found himself struggling with tremendous unease. He just could not comprehend why sometimes when things seemed to be going well for him, unexpected events would suddenly occur and disrupt his peace.

Ron stated that he initially wondered if these unwanted surprises were some form of punishment. He would find himself asking whether he did something wrong or had he neglected to do something he was supposed to do. At times, these uncertainties seemed to paralyze him.

Speaking with others often did not bring him the consolation or peace that he sought. He tried all the more to pray and offer up various mortifications, such as fasting as well as limiting or abstaining from many things that he had enjoyed in life. Despite these efforts, Ron struggled all the more wondering whether he was pleasing to God.

Ron later let me know that he had the opportunity to speak with a priest who told him not to fear anything. He pondered this for some time. This holy priest's words were those of Jesus: "... do not be afraid" (Mt 10:31). Pope John Paul II also later used these words of our Lord during his first public address as he began his pontificate. Ron said he began to realize he actually had been afraid.

As he became more and more aware of his problem, he sought further spiritual direction. Another holy priest who he encountered challenged him to thoroughly examine what was holding him back. Ron let me know that this was the most difficult thing that he had to do. He felt that the priest he was confiding in was asking him to go somewhere uncomfortable. Ron told me this must have been frustrating for the priest to handle. He was fervently trying to assist him, yet Ron did not seem to be opening up to discover the real cause of his misery. However, later in front of the Blessed Sacrament, the answer came to him. "I desire mercy, not sacrifice. Trust in Me."

Ron told me that these words of Jesus enabled him to overcome the many fears that had enslaved him. For though he had prayed and offered various sacrifices for years, he did not find true peace until he came to understand that the Lord's mercy is unfathomable and that He is a God of infinite goodness.

There is nothing we can do to earn or win God's favor. His mercy and love for us are a perfect gift that He freely offers to all. We must only be willing to receive it with heart-felt gratitude. Saint John also tells us, "There is no fear in love, but perfect love drives out fear because fear has to do with punishment, and so one who fears is not yet perfect in love" (1 John 18).

In the Most Holy Eucharist, Jesus remains with us day and night in all the tabernacles of the world. This wonderful manifestation of love has strengthened many cancer patients and provided them with a profound example of humility.

Tom was another patient I helped care for who had recognized the value of visiting our Lord in the Most Blessed Sacrament, as he himself was receiving chemotherapy for his cancer. Despite his poor health, Tom treasured being in the Lord's company. This allowed him to be present to our Divine Savior, who otherwise would have often remained alone in the tabernacle of the hospital's chapel.

We who are not ill with such a life-threatening disease should all the more frequently rush to our Lord's side in Eucharistic Adoration. In doing so we may hope to hear our Lord say to us someday, "Inherit the kingdom prepared for you from the foundation of the world. For I was ... in prison and you visited Me" (Mt 25:34-36).

CHAPTER SIX

The Transformation of Death into New Life

Families and friends of cancer patients have important roles to serve as their loved ones suffer and potentially face death. Many with such illnesses may be emotionally drained or physically weakened to such an extent that it is difficult for them to endure their conditions alone. Just as Simon the Cyrenian assisted Jesus with the cross, so, too, each of us must help others in need. Clearly, those suffering with cancer provide tremendous opportunities for families and friends to practice mercy and love.

Barb was a woman who initially had been diagnosed with breast cancer. She was a wonderful wife, mother, and grandmother. However, prior to the time her cancer was detected, she seemed disillusioned with spiritual matters. When others brought up things pertaining to religion, Barb tended to turn away, change the topic, or express a lack of faith. Yet her family members continued to pray for her. By the grace of God, she was cured of her breast cancer after receiving treatments from her doctor.

Years later, Barb contracted lung cancer. Unlike her prior breast cancer, this disease was diagnosed after having spread throughout her body. The lung cancer was expected to be fatal in the near future.

Although Barb seemed to come to terms with this difficult news, it was not clear that she had turned back to the Lord. Her cousin Elaine and her nephew Mike were particularly concerned with Barb's supposed aversion for the things of God. They prayed for the conversion of Barb's heart, so that she would recognize the Lord's unfathomable mercy and infinite love. Mike had requested prayers on her behalf from the Poor Clares of the Blessed Sacrament. These holy women prayed for Barb throughout their perpetual Eucharistic Adoration. Elaine and Mike also prayed the Chaplet of The Divine Mercy (see Part Two, Chapter Four), and they made offerings to the Marians of the Immaculate Conception, who boldly proclaim the great Divine Mercy message throughout the world. Barb and her family were thus continually prayed for through the congregation's daily Masses and prayers, including the Chaplet of The Divine Mercy.

Mike also shared with me that once when he had a bad headache, he joined this suffering to that of our Lord Jesus' suffering with his Aunt Barb in mind. Likewise, he made other offerings to the Lord to intercede for her such as fasting and abstaining from certain foods he much enjoyed. Mike later rejoiced when he learned that Barb came back to the Lord. She received the Sacrament of the Anointing of the Sick. Shortly thereafter, Barb passed from this life. The power of prayer and trust in the Lord's mercy should never be doubted. God can do all things, and He often chooses to use those nearest to us to bring about change and accomplish His holy purpose.

The Need for Change

During my specialty training in Hematology/Oncology at the University of Chicago, I had a mentor with a distinguished career, but he was dying from prostate cancer. This lovely man helped me to understand that most patients are not afraid of death, but rather they fear dying.

Death is the final end of this earthly life. However, dying is a process that may vary in its duration and degree of suffering. It is in this dying process that we see one carry his or her cross. Some embrace their crosses and join their sufferings with those of our Lord Jesus Christ during His Passion and death. This results in magnificent grace for them and in further glory for Almighty God.

Saint Faustina was a wonderful example of such an individual. She bore her sufferings from tuberculosis, mistreatment from others who often failed to understand her, and from temptations she received from the devil. Yet it was in her dying to self that she shared in the glory of God.

Saint Paul wrote, "My eager expectation and hope is that I shall not be put to shame in any way, but that with all boldness, now as always, Christ will be magnified in my body, whether by life or by death. For to me life is Christ, and death is gain" (Phil 1:20-21).

For many cancer patients, dying marks a period of great spiritual growth. In this time, they often become more aware that life is a sacred gift from Almighty God. Every moment is cherished, and things formerly taken for granted become deeply appreciated. We all, likewise, need to treasure the infinite gifts that our Lord showers upon us each day. In particular, God's mercy is a gift beyond all comprehension.

No matter how sinful our lives may have been, Jesus calls each of us to His unfathomable mercy. This provides the healing that we need. As the Second Person of the Blessed Trinity, He came to save all, not just a few. The holy Church has instructed us that Jesus is the fulfillment of the covenant, which God the Father had made with the Israelites in the Old Testament. It is He who gives hope to all and of whom the prophets of old spoke.

One such example is the prophet Ezekiel, who described a vision of a great plain filled with dry bones. He prophesied over these bones to hear the word of the Lord according to God's command. Suddenly, they were filled with spirit and came to life (see Ezek 37:1-14). Similarly, many cancer patients facing death may physically appear severely emaciated and with little life. Some of them or their family members may have had no faith in God, while others may have had a stagnant spiritual life comparable to the dead bones.

Yet as a person turns to our Lord's great mercy and love during this dying process, one truly experiences new life in the Resurrection of Jesus Christ. Our Lord tells us that He is the way, the truth, and the life (see Jn 14:6). In the eyes of the world, a person dying with cancer may only be seen as a loss of life. However, in fact, those who have remained steadfast in their faith or who have turned their lives to Christ are far more vibrant with life than many without a physical illness who lack such faith.

For many cancer patients, the dying process is a great opportunity for them and their families to center their lives on God. In doing so, they may attain the fullest life possible in both their earthly existence as well as in the age to come. Our Lord Jesus Christ tells us, "... unless a grain of wheat falls to the ground and dies, it remains just a grain of wheat; but if it dies, it produces much fruit" (Jn 12:24). We all, therefore, need to die to self as Jesus did in order to have eternal life.

Christ tells us, "Whoever wishes to come after Me must deny himself, take up his cross, and follow Me. For whoever wishes to save his life will lose it, but whoever loses his life for My sake and that of the gospel will save it. What profit is there for one to gain the whole world and forfeit his life? What could one give in exchange for his life? Whoever is ashamed of Me and of My words in this faithless and sinful generation, the Son of Man will be ashamed of when He comes in His Father's glory with the holy angels" (Mk 8:34-38). Therefore, those dying from cancer or anything else need not despair. Rather, they should rejoice by offering their lives to the Lord who, in turn, will save them.

In this vein, our Lord told St. Faustina of the great importance of the Sacrament of Reconciliation. **There the greatest miracles take place [and] are incessantly repeated. ... Were a soul like a decaying corpse so that from a human standpoint, there would be no [hope of] restoration and everything would already be lost, it is not so with God. The miracle of Divine Mercy restores that soul in full. Oh, how miserable are those who do not take advantage of the miracle of God's mercy! You will call out in vain, but it will be too late** (*Diary*, 1448).

Children often desire to someday grow up and become like their mother or father. Some perhaps wish to become a teacher, a doctor, a businessperson, and other such workers. Likewise, we all should aspire to "grow up" in spirit as well to become Jesus for the world. In praying, sacrificing, fully participating in the celebration of Holy Mass, and regularly receiving the Sacraments, one's life may be changed into that of Christ. Our lives, in turn, are then to be shared with others.

Instead of doing things merely for themselves, many cancer patients live for others. Thus, the kingdom of God becomes further established on earth. Regardless of how old, how sick, or how near death one may be, this process of formation is ongoing until we are fashioned into what the Lord wants us to be. Thus, patients with cancer should not despair but rather rejoice as the merciful Lord works in their lives. Saint Paul's words become clear to such souls as he wrote, "So whoever is in Christ is a new creation: the old things have passed away; behold, new things have come" (2 Cor 5:17).

As I completed my Hematology/Oncology fellowship and later sought a faculty position, I had the opportunity to pay a visit to the chapel of the hospital where I was interviewing. While I prayed in front of the tabernacle, the hospital chaplain, Fr. Vincent, came by, and we spoke for a few minutes. He then gave me a blessing. I later realized that this priest had been a former associate pastor at St. Columbkille's Catholic Church in Parma, Ohio, which was my home parish, where I had grown up many years before.

During the first few years that I worked in my new position, I had the privilege to witness this holy priest spread the Gospel message to patients, their families, and other visitors. He was a channel of our Lord's mercy as he visited innumerable patients and offered them the holy Sacraments of Reconciliation, Holy Eucharist, and Anointing of the Sick. After each daily Mass, Fr. Vincent extended the offering of the Anointing of the Sick not only to patients but to everyone else undergoing the stress of having a loved one sick in the hospital.

Father Vincent also preached the message of Divine Mercy by reminding us to treat everyone with respect. In particular, he had a special concern for the many support staff in the hospital. He said that they were like St. Joseph, laboring daily without notice. He said these "Josephs" were indispensable for the success of the institution, for without them, the hospital could not run. This included those who cleaned the floors, put clean linens on beds, those who transported patients, and the many volunteers who gave of their time and talent. Father Vincent preached that as we passed these individuals in the hall, we should always look them in the eye, smile, and say hello. For in doing so, we, too, may spread the Lord's kingdom by treating them as we would Christ Jesus.

As time passed, Fr. Vincent gradually slowed down. He was then found to have a type of lung cancer himself, for which he underwent treatment. He progressively declined and could no longer say Mass nor make his rounds throughout the busy hospital floors. Although he eventually passed from this earthly life, the Spirit of the Lord flourished all the more as many Eucharistic ministers and a new hospital chaplain carried on his holy work of bringing the message of mercy to the world.

Patients with cancer often fear the stigma of being diagnosed with a disease that may be fatal, yet one must remember that everyone's mortal body will eventually die. Many other forms of death are quite sudden such as that from an accident or a heart attack. However, cancer patients may often be blessed with more time from their diagnoses until death than others who pass suddenly from different causes. During this period, they may repent of their sins, restore broken relationships, and tell loved ones how much they mean to them. Most importantly, though, they can completely put their lives into God's hands, trusting in His unfathomable mercy and infinite goodness.

Jesus told us the parable of the mustard seed, which starts as the smallest of seeds, but then grows into a large bush within which the birds may build their nests (see Mt 13:31-32). Those patients who are receptive to the graces from Almighty God open their hearts and allow Him to likewise radically change them into a new creation that helps make His kingdom manifest on earth.

Jesus rebuked some Pharisees during His public life on earth for their hypocrisy in cleansing the outside of the cup while leaving the inside full of filth (see Mt 23:25). We, too, must reform our lives and repent of a similar lack of sincerity in our interactions with others. Cancer patients facing death are no longer concerned with external appearances. There is often no worry about clothes, for they commonly may only be wearing a hospital gown. Likewise, many do not focus on what make-up to put on or how their hair appears, for many of them have lost their hair after chemotherapy. When a person stops focusing on "me" and takes time to show concern for others, he or she is no longer centered on self-love.

It often amazes me when patients who are sick with a deadly cancer take the time to ask me how my family and I are doing. At night, some of them encourage me to get home to my family rather than worry about them. This genuine concern for others that so many patients demonstrate despite their own illness is a wonderful reflection of Christ's love.

The Lord's transforming Divine Mercy is very prevalent in the lives of many cancer patients. I cared for a young man named Paul, who had been diagnosed with an acute leukemia. Although he initially did well with his therapy, Paul later decided to stop treatment and not pursue follow-up medical care. He followed his own judgment and instincts.

Unfortunately, Paul's leukemia later relapsed, and he then required even more intense chemotherapy and ultimately a bone marrow transplant. His treatment was complicated by many things, including multiple life-threatening infections due to his profoundly suppressed immune system. He spent most of the last year of his life either hospitalized on the bone marrow transplant unit or at a long-term nursing care facility.

Through this period of trial, Paul's outlook on life dramatically changed. He first developed a deep appreciation for his caregivers. Although he was illiterate, he would buy thank you cards for them and do his best to sign his name. The little money he had, which was previously often spent on cigarettes, was also used to buy donuts for the healthcare providers taking care of him. His gracious efforts in spending the little he had on others reminded me of the poor widow Jesus told his disciples to observe. We hear that she gave two small coins to the Temple treasury. Jesus told His disciples that she gave more than all the others who contributed large sums of money from their surplus wealth. For the poor widow had given all that she had to live on (see Mk 12:41-44).

Furthermore, Paul witnessed to Christ tremendously with his courteous and appreciative manner as he accepted extreme suffering. Many times, he seemingly appeared abandoned by his family, and he displayed weakness in the eyes of the world. However, Paul deeply touched the lives of many as he helped draw much good out of others around him, including nurses, doctors, cleaning staff, and hospital aides.

Jesus performed many spectacular miracles during His public life on earth. Some of the most profound were His restoring life to those who had died. This included His miracle for Jairus's daughter as well as the raising of Lazarus from the dead, by which many came to have faith in Him (see Mk 5:22-24, 35-43; see Jn 11:1-44). Our Lord instructed others to remove the stone from Lazarus's tomb, so he could come to new life. We are reminded that Jesus also asks each of us to remove the stones that keep us in tombs and prevent us from having new life. These stones may be fear, despair, doubt, or some other vice. Yet when we obey the Lord, we have life to the fullest.

As wonderful as the miracles were that Jesus performed, it is important to remember that those individuals whom He had raised to life still eventually experienced the death of their physical bodies. Similarly, all cancer patients who are cured of their malignancies sooner or later pass from this life. However, by receiving new life after a cure, many have realized that this was a wonderful blessing from Almighty God. Their cures were recognized as an opportunity that enabled them to repent from past sins and to further work in this world to help build up the Lord's kingdom.

Cancer survivors have been wonderful examples of new life. They bring about incredible hope and inspiration for others who are carrying their crosses in the world. However, many such survivors have endured much suffering and turmoil in life as they received their cancer therapies. Many of them have faced death with life-threatening events such as bleeding, infections, or toxicity to various organs in their bodies. As they recover from these physical insults, many are transformed from this condition of near death to vibrant life.

Their lives may be similar to the metamorphosis from a cold, barren winter to a fresh, new spring. During this process, they undoubtedly change, and some parts of their former lives are left behind as they progress to newer states of existence.

Jeff was a man with a blood cancer who previously had a hard life. He had used illicit drugs. Later, his wife left him. When Jeff came to me, his disease had progressed to the point of imminent death if left untreated.

However, after receiving intense chemotherapy while hospitalized for a month, he achieved a remission from his disease. During this time, Jeff developed fevers. He lost his long hair and beard that he greatly loved, but with time, he learned that his external appearance was inconsequential. His goal was to be cured from leukemia. With great determination, he received cycle after cycle of chemotherapy. With each course of therapy, Jeff encountered many difficulties. Yet, after his treatment was completed, he was cured of his cancer.

While hospitalized for months of treatment, Jeff experienced love and mercy from others who cared for him. This, in turn, dramatically changed his life. He began to pray regularly, and then he tried to return the mercy that he had received to others in need.

As he followed up with me over the years, it became readily apparent that Jeff was quite a different person compared to the man whom I initially met at the time his leukemia was diagnosed. He had a great appreciation for all of his former caregivers, and he regularly visited the oncology wards to say hello to them. In addition, he sought out other cancer patients as they underwent treatment. Jeff then spent time with them in order to provide them with the encouragement and hope that he had received.

He would particularly seek out those with newly diagnosed cancers, who often were in shock or terrified. Jeff spoke with them at length of his own personal experience with such a disease. He shared with them the difficulties and fears that he had encountered. By making this time for others, Jeff's new life allowed him to do things he may never have dreamed possible.

He was able to bring God's mercy and love to many others in great need.

It has been said that the Lord works in mysterious ways. He often uses those who are weak or outcasts in the world to shame the proud and arrogant. These repentant souls are the means by which Almighty God is transforming the world with His mercy and love.

Blessed Mother Teresa of Calcutta said we are to be the hands and feet of Jesus (Mother Teresa, *Loving Jesus*, St. Anthony Messenger Press, Cincinnati, Ohio, 1991, p.79). Thus, cancer survivors like Jeff may inspire each of us to become Jesus' face and voice in the world.

Cancer patients whose lives are reflections of God's goodness, mercy, and love are like the good trees that Jesus referred to in the Gospel. Our Lord tells us, "Beware of false prophets, who come to you in sheep's clothing, but underneath are ravenous wolves. By their fruits you will know them. ... every good tree bears good fruit, and a rotten tree bears bad fruit. A good tree cannot bear bad fruit, nor can a rotten tree bear good fruit. Every tree that does not bear good fruit will be cut down and thrown into the fire. So by their fruits you will know them" (Mt 7:15-20). Therefore, even if holy people sick with cancer appear physically weak and debilitated, their lives may be spiritually rich and full of grace. Such good fruit can be recognized as the result of the Lord's life radiating through them.

Those with cancer may bear remarkable fruit for the Lord despite their illnesses by allowing His words to abide in their hearts and His Holy Spirit to work in their lives. One young couple faced great adversity when the wife, Mindy, developed an aggressive cancer. At first, Mindy was naturally petrified. At her initial visit with me, she could not even sit and talk due to her deep sorrow with tears pouring down her face. Mindy tried to meet with various people for counseling and support, but it was still extremely difficult for her to cope with her disease.

She and her husband, Tom, were young, and her mother remained overly involved in their lives. This brought added stress to the couple, particularly as Mindy struggled with her cancer. With time, Mindy received chemotherapy from which her cancer initially appeared to respond. However, later her disease worsened, and she required more therapy. As her condition deteriorated, she was placed on maximal life support for days while in the medical intensive care unit. Ultimately, she passed away from infection and failure of many of her organs.

Her husband, Tom, had previously not been as close to the Lord as he had hoped, but he gradually came closer and closer to God. In fact, Tom later thought about becoming a hospital chaplain from this life-changing experience. Although he suffered greatly from the loss of his wife, he saw it as an opportunity for grace. As such, Tom was able to come back to our Lord, the true Vine, who is our source of life.

The Power of the Holy Spirit

Transformation to new life occurs through the power of the Holy Spirit. We are told, "What the soul is to the human body, the Holy Spirit is to the Body of Christ, which is the Church. To this Spirit of Christ, as an invisible principle, is to be ascribed the fact that all the parts of the body are joined one with the other and with their exalted head; for the whole Spirit of Christ is in the head, the whole Spirit is in the body, and the whole Spirit is in each of the members. The Holy Spirit makes the Church the 'temple of the living God'" (*Catechism*, 797).

Therefore, each of us is to be a temple for the Holy Spirit. This is often manifested in the lives of many cancer patients. Our God provides us with the seven gifts of the Holy Spirit: fortitude, piety, fear of the Lord, counsel, knowledge, understanding, and wisdom (see *Catechism*, 1831).

Robert, one of my patients, showed me how fortitude may be lived. He had a recurrence of his cancer after being in a complete remission. With time, he became paraplegic after his disease affected his central nervous system. Sometimes Robert's family would ask about his prognosis and what to expect for him after becoming paraplegic. This frustrated Robert, yet he would calmly respond to his family by telling them not to worry. He just wanted to take one day at a time and to face the challenges of life as they were presented to him. He humbly accepted the will of God and wished to focus on the present rather than looking back to the past or ahead to the future.

Many others with cancer also learn the importance of living for the moment and not taking life for granted. Saint Faustina writes, "Only the present moment is precious to me, as the future may never enter my soul at all. It is no longer in my power to change, correct, or add to the past; ... and so, what the past has embraced I must entrust to God. ... and so, trusting in Your mercy, I walk through life like a little child, offering You each day this heart burning with love for Your greater glory" (*Diary*, 2).

Often, we become preoccupied with things that have not yet occurred. Planning is important to some degree, but when one becomes paralyzed from worries and uncertainties due to anxiety and fear of the unknown, it's usually self-destructive. Only by turning to the Lord and trusting in His mercy can we find the peace the world cannot give. Robert's illness had thus transformed his approach to living. He no longer sought mere physical pursuits. Instead, he prayed regularly and demonstrated great strength and courage from the Holy Spirit to face each new day with hope.

Other patients long for the Lord with a deep piety as the Holy Spirit transforms their lives to center on God alone. Alice was a patient who had fought her breast cancer for many months. Though physically she may have had good and bad days, her great love for the Lord enabled her to grow in holiness. Alice set her heart, mind, and soul on the Lord rather than on the passing things of this world. Her tremendous piety for God was readily transmitted to others. She treasured the celebration of Holy Mass, and she constantly encouraged others to participate whole-heartedly in this most perfect sacrifice.

Marian was a beautiful woman who was dying from a blood disease called multiple myeloma. She realized the world around her and all she encountered were wonderful gifts from Almighty God that must be treasured. Marian developed a deep appreciation for the sanctity of life and of God's creation. She demonstrated a holy fear of the Lord as she sought to live in holiness. Marian offered up her intense suffering with prayers and continued love of others.

Others with cancer have learned to be silent and follow the Holy Spirit's gift of counsel. John was one such individual. He developed an acute leukemia, but after much aggressive treatment, he was cured. As I reflected on John's times of trial in the hospital, I saw that he made time for silent prayer. Amidst all the commotion in a busy hospital, with doctors and nurses coming in and out of his room, this was probably difficult to do at times. However, John seemed to always pause and reflect. By doing so, he could be attentive to the Holy Spirit's gift of counsel, which enabled him to face each new day while overcoming many difficulties.

William was a man with coronary artery disease who was recovering well after bypass surgery. Shortly after, he was diagnosed with blood cancer. Initially, William was surprised and depressed when he heard this news. Rather than despair, though, he was quick to focus on the words of our Lord in the Holy Scriptures. For many years prior to this time, he had been a Bible scholar, and he had been blessed with a great deal of knowledge. From this fount of holiness, William drew more and more strength that gave him the courage to face the challenges of each day. Furthermore, despite his illness, he continued to share the knowledge that he received from the Lord in order to help evangelize others. This enabled William to maintain a steadfast faith during his own trials with cancer.

Some cancer patients have received a wealth of understanding to help them recognize the importance of their sufferings and to know how best they may serve the Lord despite their infirmities. Linda was a cancer survivor who came to such an understanding. This enabled her to inspire others by her courage and determination. Linda's faith equipped her to carry her cross and overcome the obstacles she encountered each day. Whether this was an infection, a hospitalization, or one of the many inconveniences that interrupted her life, Linda handled these situations with great patience and understanding. This allowed her to be a model of Christian living.

Finally, wisdom has been considered the greatest gift from the Holy Spirit. April was a woman with a recurrence of acute leukemia. She was a delightful lady, energetic, and filled with the Spirit of God. She saw the true meaning of life as she lived for others with love and selflessness. As such, she allowed Christ Jesus to reign supreme in her life and was a light to the world. The gift of wisdom enables one to use the other gifts from the Holy Spirit in the best way possible. This was true for April. She balanced these other gifts well. As others came to know April, their hearts were deeply touched, and they wanted to remain around her all the more.

A person who is so filled with the gifts of the Holy Spirit cannot contain them and keep them hidden. Such was the case for April, who readily shared them with others. This allowed God to use her as an instrument to help bring His great mercy to the world.

As April's illness progressed, she had made arrangements for a new caregiver to help her husband and her sons, who were in high school. She did not want to burden her family with her disease, and she even made her own funeral arrangements. As I spoke with April in the hospital, I reassured her that she had done far more than many who were facing death. I recommended that she focus on her own comfort and quality of life as she was enrolled in hospice.

Although she listened to me with love and understanding, it was clear that she continued her struggle to be a devoted mother for her sons. This selfless attitude has likewise been possessed by many of the saints as they tried to imitate our Lord Jesus Christ.

For many years, therapies in oncology were designed with the intention of directly killing cancer cells. Although this strategy has been effective for treating some diseases, it has not been effective in eradicating other cancers. Some more recent concepts of treating cancer involve targeting therapies to affect the microenvironment in which cancer cells reside. This approach can be compared to how certain animals or plants become extinct. For instance, if the climate or food supply of a certain geographic area in the world is sufficiently altered, it may become incompatible for life with certain species. Unfortunately, such devastation has sometimes occurred with the development of cities and industries. Over time, the natural habitats for certain creatures are eliminated or affected by pollution or other toxic substances in such a way that life is no longer possible.

Some cancer treatments have been developed that inhibit the formation or growth of new blood vessels necessary for tumors to survive. This strategy of changing the environment is quite appealing to help kill cancer cells. Likewise, such a strategy applied spiritually has been important for eliminating sin in people's lives for them to grow in holiness. Those affected by sin while dwelling in darkness must remove themselves from their sinful atmospheres for healing to occur. This may require that they avoid certain people, relationships, or other occasions of temptation that cause them to sin. With a simple change of these spiritual environments, many may come to the light and have their lives transformed.

Despite illness, patients remain precious in the eyes of Almighty God. As such, we must all have a deep respect for the sanctity of life, and there must be no consideration for euthanasia. No matter how old or how weak one with cancer may be, the Lord uses such individuals to further His kingdom on earth. Just as with infirmity, one recognizes that he or she is no longer self sufficient, so, too, one must completely rely on God.

By emptying oneself and putting everything into God's hands, it becomes clear that our Lord is accomplishing His great works, since it is impossible for us in our weaknesses to do so. Therefore, in hardships, trials, and situations that seem evil, the Lord can always bring about a greater good, since God cooperates with our free will. Many cancer patients and their families have found that such difficult circumstances have allowed them to grow considerably in their faith, hope, and love.

David was a man with a chronic leukemia who had required treatment intermittently for many years. However, after over a decade of living with his disease, it eventually transformed into a very aggressive lymphoma that had spread widely throughout his body. Over a short period of time, David failed to respond to treatment, and he progressively weakened physically. As he neared death, David became less responsive.

When I made my last visit to him in the hospital, he was barely alive. During that time, his loving wife had been at his side in a constant vigil. She spoke to him gently, telling him that I had come to see him. In that moment, David had a brief period of increased consciousness, and he took my hand as I sat by his bedside. Although physically he was dying, I felt a surge of his life that permeated the core of my being. During this encounter, he greatly lifted my spirit and further transformed my life by his great love.

Although chemotherapy has been effective for many patients who have cancer, there are often significant side effects, which can make the treatment unpleasant and difficult to complete. David's chemotherapy was not easy. As he grew weaker, it was no longer possible to give him more of these treatments. The toxicities he and others have experienced from such therapy may be considered by some to be the crosses that they must carry to glorify Almighty God. Despite the hardships that may be endured, those whose cancers respond to treatment or are cured may find these difficulties to be a *Via Dolorosa* that ultimately leads to resurrection and new life in Christ our Lord.

Many of my patients have had bone marrow transplants for otherwise incurable diseases. These usually include various blood cancers such as leukemia and lymphoma. The transplant procedure consists of administering high doses of chemotherapy with or without total body irradiation in an effort to eliminate disease from the bone marrow and other areas of the patients' bodies. However, during this therapy, the patients' normal bone marrow cells that would otherwise have produced healthy blood cells are also unintentionally destroyed as innocent bystanders. Subsequently, transplant patients receive compatible bone marrow from healthy donors in a process that is similar to giving a blood transfusion. The bone marrow cells then repopulate the transplant patient's bone marrow space, and as they grow, they eventually build up the blood counts again. This amazing procedure has cured many cancer patients of otherwise fatal diseases.

One can also compare this transplant approach with our spiritual life. The soul first needs intense preparation in order to be healed from deadly sin and to obtain eternal life. Faithfully following the Catholic way of life consists of making sacrifices, offering up our sufferings, praying steadfastly, participating in the celebration of Holy Mass, and receiving the Sacraments regularly. Furthermore, by following the instruction of the Church and the Holy Scriptures while trusting in our Lord's mercy, we can eradicate sin. As we die to self and live for Almighty God, we are transformed, and the Holy Spirit creates new life within us that is everlasting.

PART TWO

Spiritual Help for Those with Cancer

CHAPTER ONE

The Most Holy Eucharist: Our Source of Life

Nutrition is of considerable importance in oncology. Many with cancer lose their appetites and subsequently develop progressive weight loss that leads to further weakness and debilitation. For some of these people, malnutrition may even contribute to their death.

Jim presented to me with significant weight loss prior to his diagnosis of cancer. As the disease spread, it gradually caused his physical strength to decline. Foods that were once enjoyable to Jim lost their appeal. It became a tremendous task for him to consume three meals each day. At times, he was lucky if he could even eat one good meal each day. Needless to say, not only did this weaken Jim physically, but it also affected his self-esteem. He perceived that he was losing ground as he wasted away. For other patients like Jim, this may also cause them to become depressed, which compounds the problem even further.

In the spiritual life, those who are affected by mortal sin likewise are faced with a deadly disease. This leads to a failure to thrive spiritually and eventually to death if left untreated. The Lord's mercy is the only hope to restore spiritual and eternal life. However, in the state of serious sin, one tends to avoid things that provide grace, just as one with cancer often tends to avoid eating adequately. In both instances, this may lead to further weakening of the person's very being.

As Jim was cured of his cancer, he needed much time to recover his strength and regain the weight that he had lost. However, those forgiven of mortal sin may advance more readily in their recovery process as they again acquire further grace and holiness. A person who is severely malnourished may not be able to resume eating large meals quickly. In fact, often such patients can only gradually increase their portions of food over time. They are routinely instructed to take in small, frequent meals throughout the day in order to increase their overall nutritional intake.

Far beyond our limited understanding of what nutrition is required for physical health, God knows what is needed for us to grow in holiness. For some, this is accomplished with considerable time spent in deep contemplative prayer. For others, sacrifices are required to help further transform the soul. Little acts of charity and prayerful ejaculations may be the initial "small bites of food" that are required to help a soul grow in holiness. Then greater states of grace may be achieved through deeper and more perfect acts of love and mercy. These are the "full meals" needed to sustain and greatly increase one's spiritual life.

My patient, Jim, later regained his appetite. In fact, he overate, which resulted in obesity. Many with such a hearty appetite can no longer be satisfied with small meals. Likewise, those who achieve greater sanctity in life develop a ravenous appetite for more spiritual food. They become insatiable for the Word of God, acts of love and mercy, prayer, reception of the Sacraments, Eucharistic Adoration, and above all the celebration of Holy Mass. They do not become "spiritually obese" as long as they integrate the spiritual with everything else in their lives. This prevents one from falling into scrupulosity, over-zealousness, or even fanaticism.

Sacramental Communion

Our merciful Savior nourishes us throughout our journey in this life with His holy gifts. In particular, His Holy Word and Most Precious Body and Blood at Holy Mass sustain and richly provide us with all that we need until we arrive safely at home with Him. Jesus is the firm rock upon whom our faith is centered. He is the source of salvation for all who believe in Him. "For God did not destine us for wrath, but to gain salvation through our Lord Jesus Christ ..." (1 Thess 5:9).

Many cancer patients are wonderful witnesses of the Gospel with their hearts, minds, bodies, and souls focused on our Lord Jesus Christ. George was one of my older patients who had been receiving intense chemotherapy for acute leukemia. His therapy required him to be hospitalized for several weeks.

During this time, it was obvious that George's strength came completely from his Catholic faith and desire for the Holy Eucharist. Despite his illness and debilitated state, he would settle for nothing less than the opportunity to leave his hospital room and go down to an auditorium in the hospital for Sunday Mass. George's family had to take him in a wheelchair with catheters in place along with several poles for his intravenous medications. However, these things that may have been obstacles for many others or reasons why one could avoid attending Holy Mass seemed as nothing to George. His heart was focused on our Savior and His great mercy. The Holy Eucharist was the priceless treasure that George sought.

Jesus tells us the parable of a man finding a great treasure buried in a field. He then sells all that he has to purchase that field and attain the immense riches it contains (see Mt 13:44). We, too, need to give all that we have in order to fully receive our Lord God. We should seek the Lord in Holy Communion to provide us with the gift of Life, which is His very self.

The Holy Eucharist is the spiritual nourishment that our Lord graciously gives us for our journey through this life. Saint Faustina noted, "Once, I desired very much to receive Holy Communion, but I had a certain doubt, and I did not go. I suffered greatly because of this. It seemed to me that my heart would burst from the pain. When I set about my work, my heart full of bitterness, Jesus suddenly stood by me and said," **My daughter, do not omit Holy Communion unless you know well that your fall was serious; apart from this, no doubt must stop you from uniting yourself with Me in the mystery of My love. Your minor faults will disappear in My love like a piece of straw thrown into a great furnace. Know that you grieve Me much when you fail to receive Me in Holy Communion** (*Diary*, 156).

Therefore, the Lord God knows well that we need this heavenly food if we are to spiritually thrive. Those with cancer consume food to provide the nutrition necessary to maintain their lives, like anyone else. This food is digested and absorbed through the intestines and it then enters the bloodstream. As the heart beats, the blood circulates throughout the body in order to deliver this nutrition. This, in turn, allows for growth and healing. Similarly, as we receive the Holy Eucharist, the Lord may enter our heart and then nourish every part of our being.

Our life of faith as Catholics is centered on this awesome gift of our Lord Jesus Christ in the Most Holy Eucharist and in the Holy Sacrifice of the Mass. Jesus told us, "My Father gives you true bread from heaven. For the bread of God is that which comes down from heaven and gives life to the world. ... I am the bread of life; whoever comes to Me will never hunger, and whoever believes in Me will never thirst. ... For this is the will of My Father, that everyone who sees the Son and believes in Him may have eternal life, and I shall raise him [on] the last day. ... Amen, amen, I say to you, whoever believes has eternal life. ... I am the living bread that came down from heaven; whoever eats this bread will live forever; and the bread that I will give is My flesh for the life of the world. ... Amen, amen, I say to you, unless you eat the flesh of the Son of Man and drink His blood, you do not have life within you. Whoever eats My flesh and drinks My blood has eternal life, and I will raise him on the last day. For My flesh is true food and My blood is true drink. Whoever eats My flesh and drinks My blood remains in Me and I in him. Just as the living Father sent Me and I have life because of the Father, so also the one who feeds on Me will have life because of Me. This is the bread that came down from heaven" (Jn 6:32-33, 35, 40, 47, 51, 53-58).

Then, when Jesus was at the Last Supper with His Apostles, we hear, "While they were eating, He took bread, said the blessing, broke it, and gave it to them, and said, 'Take it; this is My body.' Then He took a cup, gave thanks, and gave it to them, and they all drank from it. He said to them,

'This is My blood of the covenant, that will be shed for many'"
(Mk 14:22-24). Thus, the Holy Eucharist is the heavenly food
that the Lord provides us with for our spiritual journey through
this life. It is the divine sustenance that is necessary to make us
holy and prepare us perfectly for eternal life.

As we more deeply contemplate the awesome mystery of
the Most Holy Eucharist, we are able to grow further in our
relationship with Almighty God. A book titled *7 Secrets of the
Eucharist* by Vinny Flynn (Stockbridge, Massachusetts:
MercySong, 2006) is helpful in this regard. Flynn presents
some of the sacred truths about this great Sacrament that the
Catholic Church has always treasured at the heart of our faith.

The first secret Flynn presents is that the Church believes
the words of Jesus Christ that He is truly alive in the Holy
Eucharist. The consecrated Host and Wine are no longer
inanimate objects. During the celebration of Holy Mass, the
priest acts in the person of Jesus. As he prays the words of
consecration over the bread and wine, they become Christ's
sacred Body, Blood, Soul, and Divinity. This change is called
Transubstantiation. The substance of the bread and wine are
miraculously transformed. The word "substance" refers to the
reality of an object or thing. After the consecration of the gifts
during Holy Mass, even though they still look like bread and
wine, their very essence has been changed into the person of
Jesus Christ. He who is God and Creator of the universe can do
all things. If He, therefore, told His Church that the Holy
Eucharist is His Body and Blood, then there should be no doubt.

Before Jesus' Ascension into Heaven, He reaffirmed, "I
am with you always, until the end of the age" (Mt 28:20). We
should be forever grateful for this unfathomable gift from
God, and we should always seek to be with Him by partaking
of the Eucharist throughout our lives.

The second secret is that Jesus is not alone in the Holy
Eucharist. He is God, and as the Second Person of the Most
Blessed Trinity, He is continually in union with the Father and
the Holy Spirit. Christ is also united with His Blessed Mother,
as well as the angels, saints, and all the members of His Body.

The third secret reminds us that there is only one Mass or Sacrifice. At every Mass, we enter into the reality of Christ's one holy sacrifice, which is ever-present before the Father. In each Mass, as members of His mystical Body, we enter into His perfect act of salvation for the entire world.

The fourth secret enables us to understand that there is more than one miracle occurring during the celebration of each Holy Eucharist. Our limited intellects can only begin to scratch the surface of the true meaning of Christ's great love for us in this Holy Sacrament. Yet each Eucharistic celebration may have profound effects on every person who partakes in this celebration, as well as on others.

The fifth secret allows us to recognize that when we consume the Holy Eucharist, we do not just receive. Instead, we are also to completely give ourselves to the Lord. This enables us to be united with Christ in the most intimate way possible during this life.

The sixth secret consists in realizing that each time we receive our Lord in the Holy Eucharist, it can be different depending on our attitudes. Some may receive the consecrated Bread and Wine with little or no faith. Others receive with their minds wandering as they think about insignificant things. The benefits of such communions are far less than for others who believe that they are approaching Almighty God and are about to receive Him into their souls. These individuals have come to understand that they are entering into the most intimate of unions with our Lord that is possible during this life. We should have such a deep appreciation for the Holy Mass and the Most Blessed Sacrament that we strive to make each communion with the Lord better than the prior one.

The final secret is that not only can we receive our Lord in sacramental communions when we physically consume the consecrated Bread and Wine, but we may also receive Him in spiritual communions. Although sacramental communions may be obtained daily by participating in the celebration of Holy Mass, spiritual communions may be obtained multiple times throughout the day. By setting aside brief moments, we may continually contemplate our Lord's great love for us wherever we find ourselves. Many great saints performed this holy practice. It enables us to place ourselves intimately in the Lord's presence. We then may cease living for ourselves but instead live for Jesus. This may, then, further prepare us for the transition from our earthly lives to that of eternity, where we may hope to be with Almighty God, our Merciful Savior.

Sally was a patient who had survived a prior breast cancer but later developed an acute leukemia. Through both of these illnesses, she learned how to suffer for the glory of God. During one of her hospitalizations, she developed profuse bleeding from her nose. Although at the time it was horrifying for her, she kept placing her trust in Jesus and focused on His great mercy. She told me that after the bleeding seemed to have temporarily stopped, she had received the Most Holy Eucharist from a Eucharistic minister in the hospital. Sally then described a sensation of almost immediate healing. She had no further bleeding during the remainder of her hospital stay. As she recovered in the hospital, each day she would pray for St. Faustina's intercession. By reflecting on this saint's tremendous love and devotion for Jesus in the Holy Eucharist, Sally could deepen her own faith. She also received inspiration from St. Faustina's extreme patience and love as she offered her own life as a pleasing sacrifice to God.

Eucharistic Adoration

The Church teaches us that the Holy Mass is the perfect sacrifice to Almighty God. For it is here that our Lord Jesus eternally offers Himself in atonement for all of our sins. Outside of the Mass, we can worship Christ in His Real Presence through Eucharistic Adoration. This holy practice enables one to commune with the Lord in this life as closely as possible outside of the Holy Mass.

Saint Faustina wrote, "I spend every free moment at the feet of the hidden God. He is my Master; I ask Him about everything; I speak to Him about everything. Here I obtain strength and light; here I learn everything; here I am given light on how to act toward my neighbor. ... I have enclosed myself in the tabernacle together with Jesus, my Master. He Himself drew me into the fire of living love on which everything converges" (*Diary*, 704). It is, therefore, in the most Holy Eucharist that those facing cancer as well as everyone else may find the source of all consolation, healing, and wisdom.

Such spiritual healing should be sought above all things. Many patients with cancer travel considerable distances to seek second, third, and fourth opinions regarding their diagnoses and treatment options. Some spend significant amounts of money during this process, thinking it is for their health. In many cases, it may, in fact, be a matter of life or death. In a similar manner, some souls longing for new life and healing from sin go to considerable lengths to make a pilgrimage to a distant shrine or church.

Mary was a patient who had a relapse of her blood cancer after failing two transplant procedures. She was expected to die within a few months. However, Mary was strongly determined to travel to Lourdes, France, to bathe in the holy water of the springs there and seek God's healing. At the time, I had doubts about her physical stamina and whether she had clearly thought about the risks of dying during such a journey. However, her two adult sons supported her desire, and they made the necessary travel arrangements.

At times, Mary may have struggled with uncertainty as to whether she actually had the strength to travel overseas. Yet she maintained her focus and sought to personally visit the shrine at Lourdes. Fortunately, she reached her destination, and by the grace of God, Mary was able to return safely home as well. Although her leukemia had not been eradicated, she still remained alive beyond a year after her pilgrimage. This was far better than what would have been expected if she had simply received further chemotherapy alone.

Others should know that they do not need to travel the world for such healing. For in their very own churches and chapels resides our merciful Savior Jesus Christ in the Blessed

Sacrament. He is awaiting us there and calling us day and night to commune with Him. Saint Faustina and the many great saints throughout history knew that their source of strength and holiness was derived from our Divine Savior's infinite grace, goodness, and mercy. They understood well that this radiates out upon us from the Most Blessed Sacrament.

Innumerable Eucharistic Adoration chapels are available throughout the world for the express purpose of allowing us to sit at the feet of our Lord Jesus Christ, as did His Apostles. Here, we may listen to Him speak to our hearts and souls of His unfathomable mercy and love. If only we would look and see with our eyes and listen and hear with our ears (see Mt 13:16) as Jesus speaks to us in the Most Blessed Sacrament, we would want for nothing in this world or the next.

Those who are too ill to commune with our Lord in the Most Holy Eucharist can always make a spiritual communion with Him wherever they find themselves. They may also repeat this multiple times throughout the day. Saint Josemaría Escrivá, the founder of Opus Dei, recommended making a spiritual communion by saying, "O my Jesus, I wish to receive You with all the purity, humility, and devotion with which Your Most Blessed Mother received You and with all the spirit and fervor of the saints."

It has been said that those who receive the Lord God in the Most Holy Eucharist are receiving a treasure of gold, while those receiving Him through spiritual communions are receiving a treasure of silver. Thus, many spiritual riches may be acquired by cancer patients and others through the holy practice of communing regularly with our God.

Humberto was a friend of mine who informed me that his mother had a lung cancer that had spread to her bones. As such, her disease was considered to be fatal within months. Although there were no known medical therapies that could cure her disease, Humberto greatly desired that his mother would at least not suffer. He flew to Brazil several times to visit his dying mother. He constantly sought to bring her comfort and to strengthen his other family members.

Humberto let me know that he was greatly distressed, since another family member was reluctant to ask a priest to visit their mother, so she could receive the Sacraments. This other family member seemed to think that this would only frighten their mother by suggesting her imminent death. In particular, Humberto prayed during Eucharistic Adoration for wisdom from the Lord in order to know how best to help his mother. He then came to realize that the Most Holy Eucharist was the best medicine.

Humberto immediately brought a priest to his mother. She received the Anointing of the Sick, which included Holy Communion. This provided her with the spiritual sustenance she so greatly needed for the journey from this life through death unto eternity with God. In the Most Precious Body and Blood of our Lord Jesus Christ, one receives Almighty God, who is the source of all life, healing, and strength.

The Lord Jesus tells us to remain in Him (see Jn 6:56), and we may do this by receiving Him in the Holy Eucharist. During our lives on earth, we may never be able to fathom the depth of Christ's love for us in the Most Holy Eucharist. Nonetheless, Jesus continually invites us to spend time with Him in Eucharistic Adoration and to receive Him during the Holy Mass.

This fountain of everlasting life and grace can never be exhausted. From it pours forth our Lord's mercy, as He so often communicated to His faithful servant, St. Faustina, and His Holy Catholic Church. The Lord tells us through St. Faustina, **In the Host is your power; it will defend you** (*Diary*, 616).

Tom was a man who took these words to heart as he underwent intense treatment for his aggressive cancer. Although he experienced considerable hardships during his life, he continually came to the Most Holy Eucharist as a fount of grace and strength. This enabled him to endure and overcome difficult events that threatened his life. Thankfully, he was cured of his cancer. Like many other patients, Tom had been transformed more and more through the Lord's power and love that He so generously offers to each of us in the Holy Eucharist.

In turn, Tom's great witness of faith was a wonderful example for others. As one encounters such holy souls, it is only natural to want to spend time with them. In doing so, people like Tom may help deepen our own faith. As I spoke with him at each visit, he had a sincere concern for my own wellbeing. Tom sought to get to know me better, and he was not shy to share his great faith in the Holy Eucharist. I found myself also growing in deeper faith and love for our Eucharistic Lord through his witness.

Enjoying intimate communion with God and then sharing this with others allow people like Tom to let our Lord further build up His kingdom among us. Thus, each Holy Communion that we receive should help us grow spiritually and bring us closer to God.

Though we may never know the full mystery of the Most Holy Eucharist in this life, those who are judged worthy for life everlasting will receive this knowledge from the Lord in His kingdom. As the Bread of Life, Jesus feeds us in a special way. This heavenly nourishment provides us with all that we need to advance in holiness to states of profound grace, and this intimate union with our Lord allows us to become and remain fruitful members of His Mystical Body.

CHAPTER TWO

The Sacrament of Reconciliation

Cheryl was a patient I cared for who had a severely compromised immune system after receiving chemotherapy for her cancer. Although she eventually became a cancer survivor, her treatment was challenging. She developed fevers, for which she was hospitalized to receive antibiotics. Such prompt medical intervention was necessary, since fevers in those with weakened immune systems may be a sign of a life-threatening infection. Fevers are never pleasant. They are uncomfortable and can contribute to dehydration and fatigue in those already weak from their cancers. Initially, fevers may be the only warning sign that something bad is developing.

In our spiritual lives, there may be warning signs that something is wrong. We need to be aware that such signs may help us recognize sin in our lives. Sometimes these may include a sense of unease after doing something wrong or encountering others' disapproval of one's sinful actions. Just as Cheryl quickly sought medical attention after having fevers, sinners must rapidly repent upon recognizing their sins. They then may seek healing through the Sacrament of Reconciliation.

Recognizing Sin and the Need for Forgiveness

We hear the Lord's call for repentance through the Sacred Scriptures that tell us, "As I live, says the Lord God, I swear I take no pleasure in the death of the wicked man, but rather in the wicked man's conversion, that he may live. Turn, turn from your evil ways! Why should you die ..." (Ezek 33:11). Further, St. Peter wrote, "The Lord does not delay His promise, as some regard 'delay,' but He is patient with you, not wishing that any should perish but that all should come to repentance" (2 Pet 3:9). Saint Paul said of God's plan to show mercy and forgiveness, "For God delivered all to disobedience, that He might have mercy upon all" (Rom 11:32).

In oncology as in other areas of medicine, genetics has become an important consideration when approaching different diseases. The genetic code contained within the cells of our bodies provides the framework of how we develop physically from conception through the remainder of our lives. Genetics is incredibly complex. By considering the vast number of genes in any one person, we can begin to appreciate the Lord's magnificent creative work as He fashions each of us into who we are meant to be.

For many types of cancer, various genetic abnormalities may occur that are unique for each disease process. Some of these abnormalities are only found in certain types of tumors, such as in lung cancer but not in breast cancer. However, other genetic changes may be common among several different cancers.

The development of genetic technology has helped better assess many patients' prognoses with specific cancers. For instance, there are many subtypes of acute leukemia that are categorized based upon their genetic abnormalities. Some of these aberrations may predict for more favorable prognoses with treatment than for those observed in other types of leukemia with normal genes. Alternatively, other genetic defects indicate that a patient's leukemia may be highly aggressive and incurable with conventional treatments. Patients with such diseases are often considered for more intense therapy such as blood or bone marrow transplantation, while others may be offered investigational therapies.

As genetic technology advanced, it became possible to assess thousands of genes within tumors from individual patients. Although many genes are present in a cancer cell or in a normal cell, not all of them are expressed. For genes to be expressed, they must be functional, and this is determined by whether they make substances known as proteins. These proteins help give a person (or a cancer) their physical composition and help regulate the metabolism.

Genetic technology has enabled physicians and researchers to determine which genes are over-expressed or under-expressed within certain types of cancers. Further knowledge of these genetic profiles may allow better treatments to be developed that specifically target these genetic abnormalities.

By considering the tremendous complexity of our genetic composition and the diverse abnormalities that may arise, one can only remain in awe of the omnipotence of Almighty God. Although seemingly vast, human knowledge of our physical beings is finite. It does not even begin to scratch the surface of who we are called to be. Only the Lord can help us come to know this reality. We were created in God's image to share in the life of the Holy Trinity for all eternity. By such design, we can grow spiritually from conception and birth through childhood and adolescence into adulthood.

As cancer may occur from genetic abnormalities that disturb normal development, our spiritual growth may also be impaired when we allow "spiritual abnormalities" called sin to affect our lives. As genetic testing may be helpful to better characterize cancers in order to treat them, we likewise need a spiritual approach to assess the soul's state of health. This is accomplished through a thorough examination of conscience and the Sacrament of Reconciliation.

Thus, cancer patients often have to contend with another battlefront besides their physical ailments. Like everyone else, they must come to recognize that this greater conflict involves confrontation of sin in one's life. In recognizing the need for Reconciliation, we have to first acknowledge that each of us commits sins. Pope John Paul II stated that one of the biggest problems in the world is the loss of any sense of sin. Many may live without ever considering that they have committed sins. It is, therefore, imperative that everyone develops a well-formed conscience. Things that are morally wrong need to be recognized as offenses against God, our loving Father.

The Sacrament of Baptism initiates one into the life of Christ and cleanses one of all sin. However, our sinful human nature causes us to fall from grace, so the Lord also gave us the Sacrament of Reconciliation. Here, we may receive the Lord's forgiveness and healing throughout our lives. After Jesus' Resurrection, He told His disciples, "Receive the Holy Spirit. Whose sins you forgive are forgiven them, and whose sins you retain are retained" (Jn 20:22-23). We also hear that Jesus "... summoned His twelve disciples and gave them authority over unclean spirits to drive them out and to cure every disease and every illness" (Mt 10:1).

Thus, as Jesus instituted the priesthood of the Church, He founded it upon His twelve Apostles. This power over unclean spirits and for curing infirmities has been passed on from the Apostles to all subsequent popes, bishops, and priests to continue healing from sin. Jesus did not give His disciples authority to only cure a few things but rather "every disease and every illness" (Mt 10:1). Thus, the Lord is present in His priests. They are the channels through which Divine Mercy flows in this great Sacrament of healing.

Some marvel at the successes of the healthcare profession, including oncology, when various diseases are cured by the grace of God. Yet, once again, physical cures are transient. Sooner or later, each of us will pass from this life. However, it is sin that threatens our eternal destiny. Our Lord ,therefore, gave us the great Sacrament of Reconciliation to free us completely from the bondage of sin. Through His holy priests, Jesus acts to cure every disease. Although physical healings are sometimes granted, spiritual healing is always possible for those who approach this Sacrament with great humility and trust.

The Act of Confession

Our Lord Jesus Christ works through His holy priests to impart forgiveness and provide grace. As a penitent soul seeks such healing, the priest helps the person discern what types of sins he or she has committed and what the best penance is for that person. This allows the penitent's soul to be strengthened in order to prevent recurrences of the sin and to bring about healing.

Such restoration to health may be likened to that from an oncologist who assesses a patient with cancer. First, the physician must confirm what type of cancer a patient has and then the extent of the disease before prescribing a specific course of treatment. Although an oncologist may see many different forms of cancer, a priest encounters "illnesses" of much greater magnitude. These abnormal spiritual conditions threaten not only a person's life on earth but also his or her soul's eternal destiny.

However, the Lord in His infinite goodness and Divine Mercy can restore everyone to perfect health when they repent and approach Him with complete trust. If only souls would not doubt but rather humbly come to our Lord, they would then fully experience His unfathomable goodness, love, and mercy, which He so freely offers to all. Jesus clearly reminds us of this through His Gospel message, as well as from His message of mercy that He entrusted St. Faustina to record for the world.

Jesus told St. Faustina, **Daughter, when you go to confession, to this fountain of My mercy, the Blood and Water which came forth from My Heart always flows down upon your soul and ennobles it. Every time you go to confession, immerse yourself entirely in My mercy, with great trust, so that I may pour the bounty of My grace upon your soul. When you approach the confessional, know this, that I Myself am waiting there for you. I am only hidden by the priest, but I Myself act in your soul. Here the misery of the soul meets the God of mercy. Tell souls that from this fount of mercy souls draw graces solely with the vessel of trust. If their trust is great, there is no limit to My generosity. The torrents of grace inundate humble souls. The proud remain always in poverty and misery, because My grace turns away from them to humble souls** (*Diary*, 1602).

One of the most beautiful parables of Jesus that illustrates Divine Mercy is that of the Prodigal Son. Anyone, no matter how great a sinner, can clearly rejoice in knowing that we have such a great God of infinite goodness and mercy.

Jesus tells us, "A man had two sons, and the younger said to his father, 'Father, give me the share of your estate that should come to me.' So the father divided the property between them. After a few days, the younger son collected all his belongings and set off to a distant country where he squandered his inheritance on a life of dissipation. When he had freely spent everything, a severe famine struck that country, and he found himself in dire need. So he hired himself out to one of the local citizens who sent him to his farm to tend the swine. And he longed to eat his fill of the pods on which the swine fed, but nobody gave him any. Coming to his senses he thought, 'How many of my father's hired workers have more than enough to eat, but here am I, dying from hunger. I shall get up and go to my father and I shall say to him, 'Father, I have sinned against heaven and against you. I no longer deserve to be called your son; treat me as you would treat one of your hired workers.' So he got up and went back to his father. While he was still a long way off, his father caught sight of him, and was filled with compassion. He ran to his son, embraced him and kissed him. His son said to him, 'Father, I have sinned against heaven and against you; I no longer deserve to be called your son.' But his father ordered his servants, 'Quickly bring the finest robe and put it on him; put a ring on his finger and sandals on his feet. Take the fatted calf and slaughter it. Then let us celebrate with a feast, because this son of mine was dead, and has come to life again; he was lost, and has been found.' Then the celebration began.

"Now the older son had been out in the field and, on his way back, as he neared the house, he heard the sound of music and dancing. He called one of the servants and asked what this might mean. The servant said to him, 'Your brother has returned and your father has slaughtered the fattened calf because he has him back safe and sound.' He became angry, and when he refused to enter the house, his father came out and pleaded with him. He said to his father in reply, 'Look, all these years I served you and not once did I disobey your orders; yet you never gave me even a young goat to feast on with my friends. But when your son returns who swallowed up your property with prostitutes, for him you slaughter the fattened calf.' He said to him, 'My son, you are here with me always; everything I have is yours. But now we must celebrate and rejoice, because your brother was dead and has come to life again; he was lost and has been found'" (Lk 15:11-32).

This great lesson from the Lord also perfectly exemplifies how one should approach the Sacrament of Reconciliation. First, the Prodigal Son came to recognize the gravity of his sin. He had rejected his loving father, removed himself from the family, and wasted everything his father had given him. By committing sin, we likewise willingly separate ourselves from God and His family.

Next, as the Prodigal Son repents from his sins, he declares that he had sinned against heaven and his father. Prior to receiving the Sacrament of Reconciliation, we should also thoroughly examine our own consciences in order to repent from all the sins that we have committed.

The lost son in the parable then returns to his father and confesses his sins. After properly preparing ourselves, we must confess our sins to a priest, who is a spiritual father to us and who, in the person of Christ, absolves us of our sins. All known mortal or grave sins must be confessed. Less serious sins should also be confessed to the priest.

During this time, our hearts should be contrite and humble, like that of the Prodigal Son, filled with sincere sorrow for all that we have done wrong. The son in the parable then said that he no longer deserved to be called his father's son. He felt that he should be treated as no more than one of the hired workers outside of the family. Likewise, in the Sacrament of Reconciliation, we also need to make an act of contrition. This has been defined as sorrow of the soul and detestation for sin, together with the resolution not to sin again (see *Catechism*, 1451).

The father in the parable then went far beyond merely offering his son forgiveness. He immediately accepted him back into his family, giving him a place of high honor and

114 | Divine Mercy, Triumph over Cancer

celebrating with great joy. Similarly, at the close of the Sacrament after the penitent receives a penance for atonement of sins, the priest grants him or her absolution. It is then that the floodgates of grace are opened. The penitent is immersed in this grace, and full healing is obtained along with the penitent's restoration to the family of God.

We also learn from this great parable of mercy that the father not only welcomes back his wayward son. He persistently calls back his older son, too, who had remained outside the house refusing to enter the celebration for his brother. Sometimes as cancer patients face terminal illnesses or other extreme difficulties, it may be tempting for them to complain about others or hold resentments against those by whom they have been offended.

However, as in the parable, our heavenly Father calls all of us into His house. There, we are to rejoice with Him since those who were dead have come to life again. God has already established His kingdom here on earth through the Passion, death, and Resurrection of our Lord Jesus Christ. As He has shown mercy and love to all, each of us is also called to do the same.

Joe was a man born into the Catholic faith. His parents were devout Catholics and actively lived their faith. However, as Joe grew older, he no longer practiced his faith. He later married and continued to follow a secular lifestyle. He developed a blood cancer while he was in his 40s. Despite having been a strong man physically, his condition gradually weakened him. Eventually, Joe could no longer work, and he became more and more dependent upon others.

During the course of his disease, Joe needed to have his spleen removed, since his platelet count was extremely low and it had not improved with other treatments. Although a normal spleen size is up to 12 centimeters, Joe's spleen was considerably larger. An enlarged spleen can act much like a big sponge or a net that sequesters and consumes platelets from the bloodstream. Many patients with enlarged spleens may have a sufficient number of platelets in their bodies, but their platelet counts in the blood can be exceedingly low. As such, these patients like Joe are at great risk of bleeding, which can be fatal. By removing an enlarged spleen, this reservoir that had been sequestering platelets from the bloodstream is no longer present, and many patients' platelet counts will subsequently improve.

Unfortunately, after Joe's spleen was removed, his platelet count did not improve. This was disappointing for him and the medical team. A decision was later made to proceed with a bone marrow transplant, since Joe's cancer had progressed and his blood counts had become dangerously low. He was then hospitalized for more than a month to undergo this procedure. During this time, his life was sustained by blood and platelet transfusions that were administered around the clock. He also received many antibiotics and antifungal medications. Joe began to bleed profusely from his urinary tract. Despite receiving more transfusions and other supportive care, his medical condition worsened.

During this time, Joe recognized he would not live much longer. His parents then came from far away to spend time with him. In particular, they continually prayed for their son and hoped he would return to the Lord. Joe's parents regularly went to Holy Mass, including at the chapel in the hospital where he had been receiving his medical care.

I later had a chance to speak to Joe's parents in private. They told me that their son had had a conversion of heart and called for a priest. He then received the Sacraments of Reconciliation and Anointing of the sick.

With his sins forgiven, Joe received the healing that he so greatly desired for such a long time. He seemed full of courage and no longer afraid of death. As he died, I reflected on Joe's conversion and how this prodigal son's return was a great cause of celebration in the kingdom of God.

Through the help of a priest in the Sacrament of Reconciliation, souls may, therefore, effectively have sin spiritually dissected out of them. With a careful examination of conscience, the penitent may allow the confessor to home in on and target each sin that is affecting his or her soul.

The priest is like a skillful surgeon who first takes a careful history from a patient in order to best plan his approach to treat the disease and restore the patient's health. The surgeon next removes the tumor, taking special care to make appropriately wide surgical margins to "get it all out." As the wound is sutured together, it gradually heals. Eventually, there may be no sign of the lesion at all. So after a good confession, with subsequent eradication of sin, a soul may also finally be healed of the affliction that threatened its spiritual life.

However, after surgical resection for some cancers, there is a need to administer chemotherapy and/or radiation therapy in an effort to kill any residual areas of microscopic disease that may have been left behind. Without such therapy, the patient's disease will eventually relapse as the residual cancer cells grow back over time.

Mary was a woman whom I cared for with breast cancer. She initially had her tumor removed, but due to the size of the lesion and the involvement of some lymph nodes under her arm, she required months of chemotherapy and radiation therapy.

Furthermore, this treatment was not easy to undergo. Mary had many side effects including nausea, vomiting, fatigue, and the loss of her hair, yet she was determined to fight her disease. Mary's courage enabled her to follow through with each treatment to save her life. She learned to take one day at a time. Such patience and trust in her care-givers allowed Mary to receive the healing that she so desired.

After a priest absolves a penitent's sins, he gives a penance in order to make atonement and reparation for the transgressions. Like chemotherapy or radiation therapy administered after resection of a tumor, the penance allows eradication of imperfections and evil tendencies deep down in a soul that would otherwise be enabled to grow back in time. Such sins that recur may be more difficult to completely eradicate, like cancers that come back after much prior treatment. However, our Lord Jesus is our Divine Physician, and His unfathomable mercy can forgive any sin and restore to perfect health all who repent and completely trust in Him.

Spiritual Direction

Spiritual direction is the means by which the Lord may use others to help form us into the people He desires us to be. G. Barrette examined this process in an article titled, "Spiritual Direction in the Roman Catholic Tradition" (*Journal of Psychology and Theology* Vol. 30(4), 2002). Barrette defined Christian spiritual direction as "the help or guidance that a person (directee) seeks and another (director) gives over a period of time in the process of growing in a loving relationship with God. This process unfolds under the continual impulse, inspiration, and action of the Holy Spirit."

There are different ways spiritual direction may come to a person. On one level, a person's family or close friends may offer assistance in this matter. Alternatively, some excellent written works as well as fine audio or video presentations may be useful. However, spiritual direction is best accomplished when one establishes a close relationship with another trained to give this important guidance.

By entering such a relationship, one may hear the Lord speaking to him or her intimately. Here, one may share the secrets of his or her soul. The spiritual director should be of high moral integrity and trained to direct souls in a confidential manner. A priest is often an ideal person to serve in this role, although it can be a layperson. However, as spiritual direction helps people examine their lives, it enables them to recognize their faults and shortcomings. This, in turn, allows them to prepare well for the Sacrament of Reconciliation.

In addition to obtaining forgiveness for our sins, the Sacrament of Reconciliation also provides us with the opportunity for spiritual direction. It is here that one may receive the help necessary to form a good conscience. The Lord uses His holy priests to grant souls special insights that best lead them along His way.

The Lord in His infinite wisdom does not leave us alone on our journey through life. In order to transform our lives, He has us encounter many different souls. Of particular importance, though, is spiritual direction.

Jesus told St. Faustina: **I Myself am your Director; I was, I am, and I will be. And since you asked for visible help, I chose and gave you a director even before you had asked, for My work required this. Know that the faults you commit against him wound My Heart. Be especially on your guard against self-willfulness; even the smallest thing should bear the seal of obedience** (*Diary*, 362). Cancer patients may likewise gain immense benefit from establishing close relationships with their own spiritual directors, who may guide them as they come to terms with their illnesses.

Saint Faustina also noted that for souls to strive for sanctity and to be fruitful, they must approach confession with sincerity and openness, in a spirit of humility and obedience. She wrote, "A soul does not benefit as it should from the sacrament of confession if it is not humble. Pride keeps it in darkness. The soul neither knows how, nor is it willing, to probe with precision the depths of its own misery. It puts on a mask and avoids everything that might bring it recovery" (*Diary*, 113).

However, many individuals with cancer have developed a humble spirit, and their compliance and docility allow them to benefit greatly from spiritual direction. It is these souls that progress readily in the spiritual life toward perfection.

Michael was a man I came to know well in oncology, who frequently received such spiritual direction. One practice he particularly cherished was taught to him by holy priests. He recalled how they instructed him to examine his conscience regularly while reflecting on the Ten Commandments of God.

Michael let me know that before his confessions, he tried to review how well he did following each of these commandments. Sometimes, he felt that he was making progress in certain areas of his life, but in other areas, he knew he needed more work. As humbling as this practice was for Michael, he told me that it enabled him to grow spiritually along the path to holiness.

Here is how he used the Ten Commandments:

1) I am the Lord your God: you shall not have strange gods before Me. With these words in mind, Michael recognized that when we put anything before God in our lives, we sin. This need not be a golden calf as for the Israelites during their exodus from Egypt. By having higher regard for anyone, anything, or any place than for Almighty God, one in essence places other gods before the Lord. Cancer patients may realize this offense if they find themselves treasuring some person in their life such as a family member or a physician above God.

2) You shall not take the name of the Lord, your God in vain. Here, Michael recalled the great necessity to honor the name of God. As such, some with cancer have taken special care not to use the Lord's name as part of swearing, even when disappointed or angered due to their medical condition. Instead, many say the Lord's name with great respect as an offering of praise and love to God.

3) Remember to keep holy the Lord's Day. Michael learned over time that we must all strive to distinguish the Lord's Day from the other days of the week. He tried earnestly to avoid all unnecessary work and use this time to grow in his relationship with the Lord and his family. Often cancer patients and their loved ones recognize the great importance of this command. Many of these individuals whom I have come to know make time to worship God at Holy Mass every Sunday despite their physical limitations. They pray and spend time with their families and friends in the Spirit of Christ.

4) Honor your father and your mother. Michael loved his parents dearly, but at times he found this to be a challenge. Although he said his parents were wonderful, there were many instances when he would become impatient with them as they aged. The small things they considered important sometimes seemed insignificant to Michael and annoyed him. Yet Michael tried all the more to hold his tongue, smile, and be accepting of his parents' wishes. Despite his busy work schedule, he also made efforts to regularly call his parents and talk. Some cancer patients also may find it difficult to always honor their parents. Nonetheless, it is imperative to love and respect the parents God gave us.

I find it wonderful to see many cancer patients' children visit them regularly and help in their care. Unfortunately, some others are neglected or forgotten by their children. Regardless of their own health, cancer patients are also obliged to honor their own parents. Sometimes they may accomplish this by words or actions that express their love. Others who are too weak or infirm to assist their parents may at least respect and pray for them. Yet still other patients have parents who are deceased or whom they never knew. They may be prayed for at anytime and any place to fulfill this great command of love.

5) You shall not kill. Michael recognized that this command not only consists of avoiding homicide but also abortion, euthanasia, and any means that directly terminates another's life in this world. He said this command also means we are to avoid actions that destroy others' wellbeing. Cancer patients, like others, should not partake in gossip or slander, since this may damage others' reputations and ruin their lives.

6) You shall not commit adultery. Michael knew well that avoiding this evil is of great importance to maintain oneself in a state of purity. He also sincerely believed that following this command is necessary to preserve the sanctity of a marriage and its bonds of love between husband and wife. Those with cancer or their spouses may be tempted at times to be unfaithful. However, with the help of the Holy Spirit, they may uphold their vows to remain faithful to each other in sickness and in health.

7) You shall not steal. Michael clearly appreciated that such actions are not from above and must be repented of immediately. Cancer patients may be enticed occasionally to take what is not theirs to try and feel better. Rather than being an act of autonomy, this, too, is an offense against God. Perhaps even worse is when others wrongfully take from those suffering with cancer. Whether this is money, property, or other possessions of the sick, it is a sin that requires repentance and must be avoided.

8) You shall not bear false witness against your neighbor. Michael found that this command enabled him to honor the integrity of others, regardless of who they are in the world. He also came to recognize that gossiping and lying are occasions when such respect is not given to others. Those with cancer, like everyone else, must keep this in mind as they seek to be forgiven and grow in holiness.

9) You shall not covet your neighbor's wife. Whether or not one is ill or no longer desirable to a spouse, this command of the Lord should be revered and obeyed. Michael let me know that after pondering this further, he realized that this did not just pertain to overt actions with another's spouse. This commandment also is intended to prevent lustful thoughts from being entertained.

10) You shall not covet your neighbor's goods. Michael reflected on these words, and he came to understand that desiring or taking what belongs to others implies a lack of trust in the Lord's divine providence. Such individuals may develop a mindset that God has not given them enough. Others may consider God to be unfair in His distribution of wealth and other gifts. At times, those with cancer may also be tempted to covet what others possess. Yet by the grace of the Holy Spirit, they may avoid such sin.

Our Lord Jesus then summed up the commandments, "You shall love the Lord, your God, with all your heart, with all your soul, and with all your mind. This is the greatest and first commandment. The second is like it: You shall love your neighbor as yourself. The whole law and the prophets depend on these two commandments" (Mt 22:37-40). Michael also treasured these words from Christ. He carefully considered them as he examined his conscience before receiving the Sacrament of Reconciliation. For by such reflection on Christ's spiritual direction, he could come to know how he failed to love God and others.

Jesus also provided St. Faustina with tremendous spiritual direction as she approached the Sacrament of Penance. The Lord told her, **My daughter, just as you prepare in My presence, so also you make your confession before Me.**

The person of the priest is, for Me, only a screen. Never analyze what sort of priest it is that I am making use of; open your soul in confession as you would to Me, and I will fill it with My light (*Diary*, 1725).

Saint Faustina also teaches us the value of a good confessor. As some individuals with cancer face their illnesses, they become withdrawn and will not speak openly with others. However, St. Faustina reminds us that in the Sacrament of Reconciliation, people conversing with their confessors need humility, openness, obedience, and trust (see *Diary*, 113, 1602).

This great Sacrament of healing from the Lord enables souls to be restored to new life. By recognizing evil and sin that offends our loving Father, people may repent and be forgiven. Then, with spiritual direction, they may remain steadfast in faith and grow in holiness. In fact, we are all called to holiness and to be saints. By being freed from sin and welcoming God into our lives, His grace allows us to share in the life of the Most Holy Trinity. This reality is a great source of hope for which patients with cancer and their loved ones may always rejoice.

CHAPTER THREE

Divine Mercy Sunday

On April 30, 2000, Divine Mercy Sunday, Pope John Paul II canonized St. Faustina Kowalska and declared the Second Sunday of Easter would now be celebrated as Divine Mercy Sunday throughout the universal Church. The message of Divine Mercy from our Lord Jesus has been entrusted to the Catholic Church since its beginning. However, throughout the 1930s until St. Faustina's death in 1938, Jesus made known to her His great desire for devotion to His Divine Mercy. This great message of hope has brought many who were lost back to God.

In *Divine Mercy: A Guide from Genesis to Benedict XVI* (Marian Press, Stockbridge, Massachusetts, 2008) Robert Stackpole, STD, examines how the Lord's great gift of Divine Mercy has been evident throughout history. The Sacred Scriptures, saints, theologians, as well as Popes John Paul II and Benedict XVI have been heralds of this holy message. Divine Mercy is the only hope for the world. On its own, humanity can do nothing good. Only when souls come to the Lord in humility, with sorrow for their sins, can healing be granted.

Pope John Paul II clearly recognized the importance of Divine Mercy. Doctor Stackpole reminds us that John Paul II considered this message not merely a doctrine or a simple devotion but a personal encounter with the merciful Savior Himself. As we personally experience His forgiveness, we can, in turn, be merciful to others. By instituting Divine Mercy Sunday as a feast to be celebrated by the universal Church, Pope John Paul II desired that everyone encounter God's mercy on a personal level (see *Divine Mercy: A Guide from Genesis to Benedict XVI*, 240-1).

Saint Paul wrote, "But God, who is rich in mercy, because of the great love he had for us, even when we were dead in our transgressions, brought us to life with Christ" (Eph 2:4-5).

So, too, Jesus told St. Faustina: **I am Love and Mercy itself** (*Diary*, 1074). **My Heart overflows with great mercy for souls, and especially poor sinners. ... it is for them that the Blood and Water flowed from My Heart as from a fount overflowing with mercy** (*Diary*, 367). **My mercy is greater than your sins and those of the entire world. ... I let My Sacred Heart be pierced with a lance, thus opening wide the source of mercy for you. Come, then, with trust to draw graces from this fountain**" (*Diary*, 1485). Jesus also said, **The greater the sinner, the greater the right he has to My mercy** (*Diary*, 723). These awesome messages of hope and mercy have strengthened many souls, including those who are living with cancer.

Of greatest importance to The Divine Mercy message is Jesus' desire for the Feast of Mercy (Divine Mercy Sunday), which is the culmination of the Easter Octave. Thus, the Easter mystery of redemption is directly connected to this holy celebration of God's limitless mercy.

There are many references throughout the *Diary of St. Faustina* regarding our Lord's command to celebrate the Feast of Mercy.

In one passage, St. Faustina records Jesus saying, **My daughter, tell the whole world about My inconceivable mercy. I desire that the Feast of Mercy be a refuge and a shelter for all souls, and especially for poor sinners. On that day the very depths of My tender mercy are open. I pour out a whole ocean of graces upon those souls who approach the Fount of My Mercy. The soul that will go to Confession and receive Holy Communion shall obtain complete forgiveness of sins and punishment. On that day all the divine floodgates through which graces flow are opened. Let no soul fear to draw near to Me, even though its sins be as scarlet. My mercy is so great that no mind,** be it of man or angel, will be able to fathom it throughout all eternity. Everything that exists has come forth from the very depths of My most tender mercy. Every soul in its relation to Me will contemplate My love and mercy throughout eternity. The Feast of Mercy emerged from My very depths of tenderness. It is My desire that it be solemnly celebrated on the first Sunday after Easter. Mankind will not have peace until it turns to the Fount of My mercy (*Diary*, 699).

To prepare ourselves properly for the Feast of Mercy we are instructed to: 1) Celebrate the Feast on the Sunday after Easter; 2) sincerely repent of all our sins; 3) place our complete trust in Jesus; 4) go to confession, preferably before that Sunday; 5) receive Holy Communion on the Feast Day; 6) venerate the Image of The Divine Mercy; and 7) be merciful to others through our actions, words, and prayers (*How to Prepare for Mercy Sunday* by Fr. George W. Kosicki, CSB, and Vinny Flynn; Marian Press, Stockbridge, Massachusetts).

This great Feast of Mercy is an unfathomable source of grace from our Lord for all people. However, we once again are challenged to respond to our Lord's mercy by responding with forgiveness to others. Our Lord gave us the "Our Father" where we pray that God will "... forgive us our trespasses as we forgive those who trespass against us. ..." Immediately after Jesus gave His disciples this prayer, He told them, "If you forgive others their transgressions your heavenly Father will forgive you. But if you do not forgive others, neither will your Father forgive your transgressions" (Mt 6:14-15). Saint James also reminds us of this as he writes, "For the judgment is merciless to one who has not shown mercy; mercy triumphs over judgment" (Jas 2:13).

Cancer patients may be consoled with this message of hope. However, there remains the challenge to each of us to show mercy.

We all know that forgiveness can often be difficult. For instance, some patients I have encountered have become depressed or bitter in light of their illnesses. These negative emotions or attitudes often are directed toward others in their families. This can lead to separations or divorces. Some patients' feelings of discontent are understandable. This is particularly true when their loved ones cannot cope in order to help care for them. They do not know how to care for them at home, and they cannot move on in life to a new level in their relationship. In these settings, cancer patients are tested beyond the struggles of dealing with their diseases. Regardless, an effort to forgive is necessary for spiritual growth and eternal life.

Our Lord repeatedly reminds us of our need to reciprocate the mercy He has shown us. This is clearly presented to us as Jesus spoke of the parable of the unforgiving servant. The man had owed a huge debt that he had no way to repay. When his master had planned to sell him, his family, and all his property for payment of the debt, the servant pleaded with him and was forgiven the entire amount he owed.

However, when he came across a fellow servant who owed him a mere fraction of the debt he had been forgiven, he refused to show mercy. Instead, he had the fellow servant thrown into prison until he repaid him. When the master heard of this account from others, he summoned that servant and called him wicked for not showing mercy in return for what was shown to him. That servant was then handed over to the torturers until he paid back the entire debt (see Mt 18:21-35).

We should, therefore, celebrate this great gift of Divine Mercy daily, but especially on Divine Mercy Sunday. Our hearts and souls should, in turn, become founts of the Lord's forgiveness and love, which are to be showered upon everyone throughout the world. We may find strength to accomplish this work through veneration of the sacred image of Jesus as The Divine Mercy.

Our Lord told St. Faustina of the two rays shining forth from His Sacred Heart in the image: **The two rays denote Blood and Water. The pale ray stands for the Water [that] makes souls righteous. The red ray stands for the Blood [that] is the life of souls ... . These two rays issued forth** from the very depths of My tender mercy when My agonized Heart was opened by a lance on the Cross. These rays shield souls from the wrath of My Father. Happy is the one who will dwell in their shelter, for the just hand of God shall not lay hold of him. I desire that the first Sunday after Easter be the Feast of Mercy (*Diary*, 299).

Steve was a man with kidney cancer. Some patients with this disease may have blood in their urine, while for others there may be flank or back pain. Still others may experience weight loss, fevers, or fatigue. Many kidney cancers may be cured if they are detected early and surgically removed before they spread to other parts of the body. Once such disease disseminates, it is often fatal with time. Thankfully, Steve's kidney cancer was found early, and he was cured after his affected kidney was removed.

In the case of sin, one may also be "cured" by God's mercy if the soul seeks such spiritual healing promptly. For if one does not heed the Lord's word to seek His mercy now, while there is time to repent and be healed, he or she will face Christ as a just judge after death. The time for mercy is now. Just as Steve's life was saved by prompt recognition of his cancer and immediate action to eradicate it, so the spiritually ill may be saved if there is urgent action to eliminate sin from their lives.

In preparation for this great Feast of Mercy, the Lord also instructed St. Faustina to make the Novena to The Divine Mercy, which is to begin on Good Friday. She was told to say the Chaplet of Divine Mercy each day (see Chapter 4 – The Divine Mercy Chaplet and the Hour of Great Mercy).

Jesus said, **By this novena, I will grant every possible grace to souls** (*Diary*, 796). Jesus also stated, **I desire that during these nine days you bring souls to the fountain of My mercy, that they may draw therefrom strength and refreshment and whatever grace they need in the hardships of life, and especially at the hour of death. On each day you will bring to My Heart a different group of souls, and you will immerse them in this ocean of My mercy, and I will bring all these souls into the house of My Father.**

You will do this in this life and in the next. I will deny nothing to any soul whom you will bring to the fount of My mercy. On each day you will beg My Father, on the strength of My bitter Passion, for graces for these souls (*Diary*, 1209).

On the first day of the novena, Jesus tells us to ... bring to Me all mankind, especially all sinners, and immerse them in the ocean of My mercy. In this way you will console Me in the bitter grief into which the loss of souls plunges Me (*Diary*, 1210). Therefore, all people are called to our Lord's fount of Divine Mercy this day, since we are all sinners. We cannot hold back; we must bring everyone. Those who visit the sick physically or spiritually have an obligation to present them to the Lord. However, even those who are ill with cancer can bring others to the Lord this day. This includes their families, friends, relatives, nurses, physicians, and others that they encounter during life.

On the second day of the novena, Jesus said, **Today bring to Me the souls of priests and religious, and immerse them in My unfathomable mercy. It was they who gave Me the strength to endure My bitter Passion. Through them, as through channels, My mercy flows out upon mankind** (*Diary*, 1212). Even today, these holy priests and religious have remained the pillars of the Catholic Church. Throughout time, the suffering face of Jesus remains present in His brothers and sisters, including those with cancer. Our Lord is also present in priests and religious who help these souls carry their crosses and who strengthen them as they channel God's mercy upon them.

One patient I had the honor to care for was Fr. John, who had pancreatic cancer. This holy man embraced his cross as he received chemotherapy throughout Lent 1997. Although Fr. John died within months from the time that his cancer was diagnosed, his toil and good example will not be forgotten. Amidst the daily struggles he faced while receiving experimental treatment for his disease, he maintained great composure and peace. His strong faith in God and His providence were overtly evident.

We should always pray for our priests throughout life, for they are the shepherds the Lord has provided for us. Likewise, we should offer prayers for all religious, for God has given them to us as intercessors and models of holiness. Holy men and women like Fr. John have given their lives to Christ to help bring us to Him as our source of salvation. We, in turn, should be grateful and reciprocate with lives of obedience and love for them.

The third day of the novena brings us our Lord's desire for the faithful. He says, **Today bring to Me all devout and faithful souls, and immerse them in the ocean of My mercy. These souls brought Me consolation on the Way of the Cross. They were that drop of consolation in the midst of an ocean of bitterness** (*Diary*, 1214). Although in the world there are those who lack faith, many individuals with cancer brightly shine with a strong devotion to our Lord and His Most Blessed Mother. They stand by our Lord in His suffering as they try to carry their own much smaller crosses.

Linda was a woman who had just recovered from treatment for her aggressive blood cancer. She had incredible faith that could not be shaken by the fear of death. Rather, she actively prayed daily and placed her trust in our Lord. Even though patients like Linda trust in the Lord for physical healing, much more importantly is their confidence in Jesus' mercy for complete spiritual healing.

The Lord requests during the fourth day of the novena, **Today bring to Me those who do not believe in God and those who do not yet know Me. I was thinking also of them during My bitter Passion, and their future zeal comforted My Heart. Immerse them in the ocean of My mercy** (*Diary*, 1216). This intention from our Lord should be a cause of great rejoicing and hope. Our Savior Jesus Christ clearly and unequivocally assures us of His deep desire for every soul, regardless of its lack of faith. We are to pray and to live fervently in the Lord, the Good Shepherd, to help bring our brothers and sisters into His sheepfold.

Therefore, those with cancer who have great faith should not lose heart when contemplating their loved ones who do not believe in God. Instead, by consecrating such souls, particularly during the Novena to The Divine Mercy, and offering up their prayers and sufferings in union with the Holy Mass, they help mediate God's power to transform others.

On the fifth day of the novena, Jesus tells us, **Today bring to Me the souls of those who have separated themselves from My Church, and immerse them in the ocean of My mercy. During My bitter Passion they tore at My Body and Heart, that is, My Church. As they return to unity with the Church My wounds heal and in this way they alleviate My Passion** (*Diary*, 1218). A tremendous void may form within any family that is damaged from the estrangement of a member due to hard feelings, resentment, or isolation between individuals. The effects are not just felt by one or two members, but by the entire family. Such separations caused our Lord Jesus to suffer horribly as chunks of His sacred flesh were ripped off during His scourging at the pillar. These pieces of Christ's Body include those brothers and sisters who remove themselves from His Church.

Marty was a woman I knew who was confined to the hospital for several weeks. She told me that certain experiences changed her life. Previously, she had estranged herself from the Church. However, later Marty found that during her sufferings, others showed her great love in a spirit of faith. This caused her to seek union again with the Church. Although she later died, Marty received The Divine Mercy message. Her life had been transformed. Others with cancer also may often experience considerable challenges in family life, which may result in separation between individuals. Despite these trying circumstances, our Lord greatly desires unity to bring about the healing that is necessary. Of course, this is only possible with complete trust in God's mercy.

On the sixth day of the novena, Jesus said, **Today bring to Me the meek and humble souls and the souls of little children, and immerse them in My mercy. These souls most closely resemble My Heart. They strengthened Me during My bitter agony. I saw them as earthly Angels,** who would keep vigil at My altars. I pour out upon them whole torrents of grace. Only the humble soul is able to receive My grace. I favor humble souls with My confidence (*Diary*, 1220). Children with cancer are often among the most humble of souls and are included with those for whom we pray on this day of the Novena to The Divine Mercy. In some cases, these children have been ill all of their lives. They may consider the medical care that they continually require to be just part of their daily routine. They do not have an understanding of what not being sick is like.

Brandon was a young boy with leukemia who became adjusted to his illness. He found that coming in for blood tests and chemotherapy treatments was a normal part of his life as much as going to school, doing homework, or playing with other children. Brandon had a delightful personality, which readily caused others to fall in love with him. As I had the chance to participate in his medical care, this little boy helped teach me the true meaning of humility. He entrusted himself completely to those who cared for him. At times, I am sure that he was afraid, but when others calmly reassured him, Brandon's unease would pass rather quickly.

As one witnesses the openness with which many such children accept their crosses and carry on in life, it is humbling to adults who may not be able to cope with illnesses of much less severity. This may be a reflection of a child's ability to just trust in Jesus. Many adults may learn from these little ones by letting go of things in this world first to fully embrace our Lord's Gospel message. Obedience is another means by which one can show humility. This, too, is often exemplified in those children and adults who have the deepest trust in our Lord.

On the seventh day of the novena, Jesus requested, **Today bring to Me the souls who especially venerate and glorify My mercy, and immerse them in My mercy. These souls sorrowed most over My Passion and entered most deeply into My Spirit. They are living images of My Compassionate Heart. These souls will shine with a special brightness in the next life. Not one of them will go into the fire of hell. I shall** particularly defend each one of them at the hour of death. ... I Myself will defend as My own glory, during their lifetime, and especially at the hour of their death, those souls who will venerate My fathomless mercy (*Diary*, 1224, 1225).

This message of profound consolation should encourage all to venerate and glorify Jesus' mercy without ceasing. Many with cancer never lose hope, but rather maintain positive attitudes and trust in their caretakers. Even more, infinitely more important, is it necessary for all souls to maintain a strong faith and hope in our Lord's Word.

During the eighth day of the novena, Jesus said, **Today bring to Me the souls who are in the prison of Purgatory, and immerse them in the abyss of My mercy. Let the torrents of My Blood cool down their scorching flames. All these souls are greatly loved by Me. They are making retribution to My justice. It is in your power to bring them relief. Draw all the indulgences from the treasury of My Church and offer them on their behalf. Oh, if you only knew the torments they suffer, you would continually offer for them the alms of the spirit and pay off their debt to My justice** (*Diary*, 1226).

When one dies of cancer, we cannot assume that our work and care for them is completed. Those who require the purification of purgatory may need our prayers and sacrifices even more than when they lived their mortal lives with physical illnesses. The Holy Sacrifice of the Mass is the perfect prayer for such souls.

Other sources of indulgences that are of great value, particularly when offered in union with the Mass, include the Chaplet of The Divine Mercy, the Novena to The Divine Mercy, and the Holy Rosary. Fasting, temperance, almsgiving, as well as offering up other sacrifices and prayers, are also beneficial. By consecrating every act and work that we perform throughout the day, we may be able to greatly assist all of our brothers and sisters in purgatory. As we pray for the intercession of the angels and saints in heaven, we also invoke their aid to help the suffering souls.

Those individuals who offer up their sufferings from cancer for the sake of those in purgatory are a wonderful example to us all. They demonstrate love, which, in turn, transforms their own lives. They may share in the hope that those souls whom they have helped in purgatory will, in turn, someday help them as well, if they should require such purification after death.

On the ninth day of the novena, our Lord Jesus requested the following: **Today bring to Me souls who have become lukewarm, and immerse them in the abyss of My mercy. These souls wound My Heart most painfully. My soul suffered the most dreadful loathing in the Garden of Olives because of lukewarm souls. They were the reason I cried out: "Father, take this cup away from Me, if it be Your will." For them, the last hope of salvation is to flee to My mercy** (*Diary*, 1228). All people can potentially become complacent and, therefore, contribute to the Lord's suffering.

As those with cancer face their illnesses, some may seek self-pity, but others see this time as an opportunity for profound spiritual growth. In some cases, the families and friends of patients may distance themselves from those who are sick, and their love grows cold. They then may become the lukewarm souls that our Lord referred to on this day of the novena. In contrast, others take our Lord's words to heart and radically change their lives as they pour out love on those suffering from cancer.

Charles was a man whose sister had a lymphoma, and the only potential for cure was with a bone marrow transplant. Unfortunately, his sister's condition rapidly deteriorated, and she died before this procedure could be performed. However, Charles was moved by this experience, and he sought to donate his bone marrow to other patients in need as a way to honor his sister.

Millions of similar Good Samaritans are also enrolled in the National Marrow Donor Program registry. They freely give of their time and bone marrow to help save the lives of others. Such souls do not remain complacent when they see others in need. Instead, they are motivated by love to imitate Christ.

This message of mercy is so important that our Lord urged His priests to proclaim it throughout the world. Cancer patients may, therefore, receive tremendous graces from holy priests who bear this message as they minister to them and others in their flock.

Jesus told St. Faustina, **My daughter, do not tire of proclaiming My mercy. In this way you will refresh this Heart of Mine, which burns with a flame of pity for sinners. Tell My priests that hardened sinners will repent on hearing their words when they speak about My unfathomable mercy, about the compassion I have for them in My Heart. To priests who proclaim and extol My mercy, I will give wondrous power; I will anoint their words and touch the hearts of those to whom they will speak** (*Diary*, 1521). These words have been fulfilled in holy priests such as Pope John Paul II, the Great Mercy Pope.

Jesus explained to His disciples why He spoke to the people in parables by saying, "... knowledge of the mysteries of the kingdom of heaven has been granted to you, but to them it has not been granted. ... because 'they look but do not see and hear but do not listen or understand'" (Mt 13:11, 13). Then our Lord quoted the Prophet Isaiah saying, "Gross is the heart of this people, they will hardly hear with their ears, they have closed their eyes, lest they see with their eyes and hear with their ears and understand with their heart and be converted and I heal them" (Mt 13:15).

These words of our Lord remain relevant to all. Although God has continuously poured out His mercy as a great ocean upon us, many souls have closed their eyes, ears, and hearts to Him.

Jesus spoke about such souls to St. Faustina as He said, **There are souls who thwart My efforts** (*Diary*, 1682). ... **Souls without love and without devotion, souls full of egoism and self love, souls full of pride and arrogance, souls full of deceit and hypocrisy, lukewarm souls who have just enough warmth to keep them alive: My Heart cannot bear this. All the graces that I pour out upon them flow off them** as off the face of a rock. I cannot stand them, because they are neither good nor bad (*Diary*, 1702).

Our Lord spoke further to St. Faustina, saying, **Souls perish in spite of My bitter Passion. I am giving mankind the last hope of salvation; that is, the recourse to My Mercy** (*Diary*, 998). **If they will not adore My mercy, they will perish for all eternity. Secretary of My mercy, write, tell souls about this great mercy of Mine, because the awful day, the day of My justice, is near** (*Diary*, 965).

It is so pleasing to see many cancer patients and their families embrace this message of hope with open hearts. However, still others remain indifferent and do not see, hear, or understand the Lord's gracious words of unfathomable mercy. This holy gift may come to them in many ways, including through a priest or a religious, a lay minister, a television or radio program, an article, a pamphlet, or even through another family member or friend.

The Lord spoke through the Prophet Jeremiah in this regard as well, saying, "Cursed is the man who trusts in human beings, who seeks his strength in flesh, whose heart turns away from the Lord. He is like a barren bush in the desert that enjoys no change of season, but stands in a lava waste, a salt and empty earth" (Jer 17:5, 6). However, then Jeremiah wrote, "Blessed is the man who trusts in the Lord, whose hope is the Lord. He is like a tree planted beside the waters that stretches out its roots to the stream: It fears not the heat when it comes, its leaves stay green; in the year of drought it shows no distress, but still bears fruit" (Jer 17:7, 8).

Lois was a woman who I came to know well. Her husband had been sick and gradually declining from his cancer for years before he eventually passed from this life. Lois was exhausted by the time of her husband's death, but she let me know how much she missed him. Like so many other faithful spouses, she cherished her wedding vows "until death do us part."

One's love for others, including family members or patients, does not cease with physical death. As such, the Church has always stressed the importance of praying for the dead. This certainly is a wonderful means to further spread

The Divine Mercy message and to unite the Church Militant on earth with that of the Church Suffering in purgatory and the Church Triumphant in heaven.

As Lois reflected on her former life with her husband, she told me that she previously had made many plans. However, they often did not work out the way that she intended. Lois stated that when she recalled how God worked in her life during these instances, she was amazed. She then would say, "Wow, what a good plan the Lord accomplished for me instead." One of my parish priests also liked to say that if you would like to make God laugh, tell Him your plans.

Despite Lois's grief from the loss of her husband, she knew that she had work to do for the Lord. This started each day with her participation in the celebration of Holy Mass. Lois then spent time regularly in Eucharistic Adoration. She also was a Eucharistic minister. She visited the sick and brought Jesus to them. Lois had a tremendous devotion to The Divine Mercy of our Lord, and she had organized a special service at her parish that began at 3 p.m. every year to celebrate Divine Mercy Sunday. She led the Holy Rosary and the Chaplet of The Divine Mercy.

In addition, each year Lois's priest would have the congregation come up to individually venerate The Divine Mercy image. The priest would then read the Gospel and give a wonderful homily on The Divine Mercy message as our Lord had requested of His faithful servant, St. Faustina.

God had previously worked miracles throughout Sacred Scripture for widows. As I reflected on Lois's example, it was apparent how God's awesome message of Divine Mercy had flourished through the efforts of an older woman who trusted in Him.

CHAPTER FOUR

The Divine Mercy Chaplet and the Hour of Great Mercy

Exercise and physical therapy are important to help rehabilitate a patient who receives cancer therapy. Similarly, after sin, one loses "spiritual strength" that needs to be restored. Spiritual exercises provide the means by which souls may be strengthened for their journey to our Lord. The power of prayer cannot be underestimated as Almighty God has taught us through Holy Scripture and His holy Church. Cancer patients and their loved ones often pray continually, and this is a wonderful offering to God.

We have been taught that prayer may come in many different forms, but some broad classifications may be considered. First, we should offer prayers of adoration to the Lord for His infinite goodness and Divine Mercy, which He so freely shares with us despite our many shortcomings. Then prayers of thanksgiving are to be offered to God for everything that He has done for us previously, for all that He continues to do for us now, and for all that He will do for us in His great mercy. Throughout our lives and eternity, we could not even come close to giving God the gratitude He deserves. Prayers of atonement for our sins are appropriate to make amends for the faults that have separated us from our Lord. Finally, we may petition God for requests deep in our hearts. Throughout all forms of prayer, we should strive to grow deeper and deeper in our love for Almighty God and in our trust in His infinite mercy.

One powerful prayer is the Chaplet of The Divine Mercy, which our Lord taught St. Faustina. She had seen an angel, the executor of divine wrath, about to strike the earth in a particular place. Saint Faustina begged the angel to hold off for a few moments so the world could do penance. However, she found her plea to be nothing in the face of divine anger. Our Lord then gave her the words of the Chaplet of Divine Mercy to pray. As she did so, St. Faustina saw the angel's helplessness, and he could not carry out the punishment due for sins (see *Diary*, 474).

Jesus told her, **Oh, what great graces I will grant to souls who say this chaplet; the very depths of My tender mercy are stirred for the sake of those who say the chaplet. ... Speak to the world about My mercy; let all mankind recognize My unfathomable mercy. It is a sign for the end times; after it will come the day of justice. While there is still time, let them have recourse to the fount of My mercy; let them profit from the Blood and Water which gushed forth for them** (*Diary*, 848).

Those with cancer may receive immense graces and mercy through the recitation of the Chaplet of Divine Mercy. Our Lord told St. Faustina, **Say unceasingly the chaplet that I have taught you. Whoever will recite it will receive great mercy at the hour of death. Priests will recommend it to sinners as their last hope of salvation. Even if there were a sinner most hardened, if he were to recite this chaplet only once, he would receive grace from My infinite mercy. I desire that the whole world know My infinite mercy. I desire to grant unimaginable graces to those souls who trust in My mercy** (*Diary*, 687).

I have encountered a number of patients with life-threatening cancers who, while hospitalized, embraced this great prayer of mercy. As we begin the prayer in the Name of the Father, and of the Son, and of the Holy Spirit, we honor our Almighty Triune God.

Next, with the "Our Father," we pray to the Lord in the words our Savior Jesus taught us. This is followed by the "Hail Mary," which venerates Our Blessed Mother and invokes her powerful intercession as our merciful Mother. Then the Apostles' Creed is recited, which further unifies our prayer with that of all the Church.

Souls are then given new life with the words, "Eternal Father, I offer You the Body and Blood, Soul and Divinity of Your dearly Beloved Son, our Lord Jesus Christ, in atonement for our sins and those of the whole world" (prayed on the Our Father beads of a rosary before each decade). This is followed by the words, "For the sake of His sorrowful Passion, have mercy on us and on the whole world" (prayed on the smaller Hail Mary beads comprising each decade of a rosary). The prayer is then concluded by praying three times, "Holy God, Holy Mighty One, Holy Immortal One, have mercy on us and on the whole world" (*Diary*, 476).

Jesus told St. Faustina of the power and importance of this prayer, particularly for the dying. **At the hour of their death, I defend as My own glory every soul that will say this chaplet; or when others say it for a dying person, the indulgence is the same. When this chaplet is said by the bedside of a dying person, God's anger is placated, unfathomable mercy envelops the soul, and the very depths of My tender mercy are moved for the sake of the sorrowful Passion of My Son** (*Diary*, 811). Just as the good thief who repented while being crucified with Jesus obtained Paradise from our Lord (see Lk 23:40-43), so, too, can any soul who invokes God's mercy with a repentant heart.

Tim was a patient who I will never forget after witnessing how the healing power of prayer touched his life. Our first encounter occurred when I was responsible for covering the inpatient oncology ward at the hospital where I was working. I received a call from a physician who first evaluated Tim at another hospital, and he wished to transfer him to our institution for urgent medical care. Tim had presented with markedly abnormal blood counts, including a white blood cell count that was more than 25 times above the normal range. He also had fatigue and a diffuse rash that caused him considerable discomfort from itching.

After Tim arrived at our hospital, my inpatient team quickly ordered many tests to establish a diagnosis. This included various blood tests, CT scans, and biopsies. While awaiting the results, he was placed on a medicine to lower his elevated white blood cell count that may have otherwise been life threatening. Tim was then found to have a rare type of lymphoma, highly aggressive, and usually fatal.

During these first few days of his hospitalization, he seemed overwhelmed at times from all the medical testing he underwent and the information he was given. Nonetheless, Tim was a man of prayer with a calm demeanor. His wife was usually at his bedside offering him support as well. People prayed for Tim during this time of trial. He then received chemotherapy, and his blood counts transiently improved.

This allowed him to go home and continue his treatments as an outpatient. However, within a few months, Tim's disease rapidly worsened, and he clinically deteriorated. During this time, he lost at least 40 pounds, and he was extremely weak. Further treatment was ineffective, and since Tim was dying, he wished to go home with hospice care. Arrangements were made for him to leave the hospital. I did not expect to see him again.

All the while, people continued to pray for Tim. In particular, I prayed the Chaplet of The Divine Mercy for him. Typically, when patients are sent home with hospice, their physicians are notified by the nurses what needs they have and how they are doing. In Tim's case, I expected a call shortly after he left the hospital to let me know that he had died at home, in peace. However, as each day passed and then as weeks went by, this call never came. I was perplexed.

When I inquired how Tim was doing, his hospice nurse informed me that he was still alive and not in need of more care. After a few months, I received a message from the hospice team that Tim seemed fine, and they were discharging him from hospice care. I was dumbfounded at this news and asked to have an appointment with him in my outpatient clinic.

On the day Tim came to see me, I knocked on the exam room door where he had been waiting. I honestly had no idea what to expect. When I opened the door, I was amazed to see Tim, for his appearance had markedly changed. This man who formerly left the hospital weak and frail, unable to walk, and near death had been radically transformed. He beamed with life as he smiled at me and grasped my hand firmly. Tim had gained 40 pounds back and had all of his former strength that he possessed prior to his cancer diagnosis and perhaps even more. I was delighted to see his joyful countenance. However, I was uncertain what to tell him next.

As I sat next to him and his wife, I looked up his blood test results on a computer in the exam room. I wondered whether they would be better than they were before when I last saw him. I prayed that they would be. As I looked on the computer screen, I was elated to find that Tim's blood counts were normal.

Although I was filled with wonder and excitement, I could not honestly tell him that things were fine until he had follow-up CT scans performed. I let Tim know that I had prayed for him, and I felt many others had done so as well. He then went for his CT scans. To my great delight, there was no evidence of his lymphoma, despite him not having received any further medical treatment for many months. I had the pleasure of letting Tim and his wife know the good news, and they rejoiced with me.

He returned months later, and his blood tests and CT scans once again were still normal. His healing seemed miraculous. In my opinion, there was no medical explanation for what had transpired in Tim's life.

Tim continued to thrive, and I know that he was profoundly grateful for the gift of a second chance at life. His physical healing is a wonderful example of the power of intercessory prayer and the Chaplet of The Divine Mercy. Nevertheless, more importantly, is the spiritual healing that this powerful prayer imparts. For instance, Jesus cured a paralytic of his physical illness as an outward manifestation of the much more important healing, which was the forgiveness of his sins (see Mark 2:1-12).

Saint Faustina also recorded that Jesus said, **My daughter, encourage souls to say the chaplet which I have given to** you. It pleases Me to grant everything they ask of Me by saying the chaplet. When hardened sinners say it, I will fill their souls with peace, and the hour of their death will be a happy one.

Write this for the benefit of distressed souls; when a soul sees and realizes the gravity of its sins, when the whole abyss of the misery into which it immersed itself is displayed before its eyes, let it not despair, but with trust let it throw itself into the arms of My mercy, as a child into the arms of its beloved mother. These souls have a right of priority to My compassionate Heart, they have first access to My mercy. Tell them that no soul that has called upon My mercy has been disappointed or brought to shame. I delight particularly in a soul which has placed its trust in My goodness.

Write that when they say this chaplet in the presence of the dying, I will stand between My Father and the dying person, not as the just Judge but as the merciful Savior (*Diary*, 1541).

I have witnessed that many cancer patients, including those who have died, have received profound healing through our Lord's Chaplet of The Divine Mercy. Whether or not there is restoration to physical health, there is always spiritual healing from this great prayer. I find these prayerful experiences to be spiritually uplifting for me as well. Our Lord God may use the deaths of such patients as sources of profound grace and new life not only for them but for their families, friends, and many others. Almighty God is truly our Divine Physician. In His infinite wisdom, He knows how to best bring healing to all.

Richard was a man who I had the opportunity to get to know in oncology. His life had been radically transformed by The Divine Mercy message. Richard had developed a deep prayer life that was obvious to many who came to know him. He loved the Lord above all things. He also despised sin, for he knew that this wounded people's relationships with their loving God.

Richard had one deep desire that he shared with me. This desire was that all souls would be with the Lord in His kingdom for all eternity. The thought of even one person choosing to reject God in order to obtain hell forever completely horrified Richard. As he considered this further, it was overwhelming for him to think that any soul was capable of making this grave mistake. Yet as Richard came to know of The Divine Mercy message, his fear dissipated. He also understood that each of us has a responsibility to wisely use our free wills from God.

As Richard and I conversed, it became clear that he was aware of his limitations as one mere man. However, he was extremely confident in the omnipotence of Almighty God and in His unfathomable mercy. This trust in the Lord was strengthened over time as Richard further developed his prayer life. At the center of this prayer life was the Holy Mass and Eucharistic Adoration. This became a daily practice for him that allowed the life of Christ to permeate his soul. Richard helped others to understand the critical need of sharing the gifts that we have received from the Lord with others. He was clear that of greatest importance is sharing The Divine Mercy message.

As Richard pondered how he best could serve others, he prayed for guidance. As he spent private time with the Lord, he began praying The Divine Mercy Chaplet for souls. He recalled from St. Faustina the tremendous power this prayer had in invoking God's mercy. When he heard that a patient with cancer was dying, he prayed the Chaplet of Divine Mercy for the person. In some cases, he would make his way to the dying person's hospital room. If there were others in the room, Richard would sometimes just stand out in the hallway nearby. In other instances, he would slip out into a stairwell as a private place of prayer. Here, Richard would intercede for countless souls as they faced death. With time, this holy practice became more and more a part of his life.

Richard let me know he was also inspired by the Book of Tobit in the Old Testament. From this Sacred Scripture, he learned how Tobit would get up and leave his meal at the news of a person's death to provide them with a dignified burial (see Tob 2:4). Tobit was ridiculed for this, but God rewarded his integrity and virtue. The Lord sent His archangel, St. Raphael, to bring about healing for Tobit and a safe journey for his son, Tobiah, as he sought a wife. However, the archangel's identity was hidden during this time under the appearance of a man.

Cancer patients may likewise contemplate that our Lord sends special messengers into their lives to provide them with strength, guidance, and consolation. At the end of the book, Tobit told Tobiah to pay St. Raphael not only the agreed upon wage but also a bonus. Tobiah, in turn, offered his heavenly companion half of what he had for repayment. The archangel of God then revealed himself and informed the two that giving alms is of great value, for it expiates sin (see Tob 12:8-9). Even today, the alms offered by cancer patients and their families surely make reparation for sin.

While Richard constantly prayed for the dead and the dying, he, too, found himself being ridiculed at times, even by his family, who loved him. Instead of becoming discouraged, this strengthened his resolve all the more. He let me know that such persecution, no matter how small, may well be a sign that we are on the right track. For Jesus told us, "If they persecuted Me, they will also persecute you" (Jn 15:20).

Richard and I spoke further. He said that after he prayed the Chaplet of The Divine Mercy to intercede for the dying, he could often sense dramatic changes. For some, there appeared to be a resolution of anxiety or an improvement in their clinical condition. Others came to accept their death as the holy will of God. In other cases, he noticed family members more peacefully came to terms with their loved one's death.

In particular, Richard recalled praying much for one patient named Lou. This man was critically ill from his cancer, and he was cared for in the intensive care unit. Lou had many family members constantly with him. Richard experienced their grief and anxiety as he watched them face tremendous uncertainties as to whether or not Lou would survive each day. Just when they thought he was clinically improving, another problem would develop. Richard let me know that he had to do something.

He wished to intercede to Almighty God for Lou and his loved ones in the most powerful way possible. Therefore, he participated in the daily celebration of Holy Mass. As a direct extension of this perfect sacrifice, Richard would fervently pray the Chaplet of Divine Mercy. By invoking what Jesus suffered for souls during His sorrowful Passion and death, Richard could further partake in this perfect act of worship to Almighty God.

Whether prayed at Lou's bedside or far away, the multiple Chaplets of Divine Mercy offered by Richard were to atone for any sins that Lou had committed. Richard realized how helpless Lou had become. While on a ventilator, with a marked reduction in his level of consciousness, it was not clear whether Lou would ever be able to speak or convey his thoughts to others again. However, the Lord works in mysterious and wonderful ways in each person. Richard knew that God alone could communicate clearly with Lou. He had great trust in the power of the Chaplet of Divine Mercy, and with it, he interceded for Lou in order to assist in God's healing.

Of course, the Lord may certainly heal anyone of any infirmity by His mere will. Yet, in His infinite wisdom, He allows others to help accomplish His Divine purpose. Richard understood well that we are part of the Body of Christ. As such, we may be His hands, His face, and His voice to others. Through God's grace residing within our souls, we may, in turn, bring Christ to others.

Lou and his family received the Lord's mercy prior to his death. Although his loved ones were appropriately sorrowful as he passed from this life, they also seemed to have peace. Their faith was strengthened by this experience, and they could be comforted by the hope that Lou had a share in the Lord's Resurrection. Regardless of his former doubts, Richard came to know the importance of his intercessory prayer. We also should be open to assist others with this powerful prayer of Divine Mercy Jesus gave us.

The Lord also told St. Faustina, **At three o'clock, implore My mercy, especially for sinners; and, if only for a brief moment, immerse yourself in My Passion, particularly in My abandonment at the moment of agony. This is the hour of great mercy for the whole world. I will allow you to enter into My mortal sorrow. In this hour, I will refuse nothing to the soul that makes a request of Me in virtue of My Passion** (*Diary*, 1320).

From the infancy of the Church, spending this time in prayer has been important. For instance, we hear how St. Peter and St. John healed a crippled man through the power of Jesus' name as they were going up to the temple area for the three o'clock hour of prayer (see Acts 3:1). Many holy souls still today continue to honor the Lord at the Hour of Great Mercy.

Reginald was a man I came to know well as I worked in hematology/oncology. He greatly cherished The Divine Mercy message. It had brought him tremendous healing after he repented from living a secular lifestyle. Reginald tried every day to take time at the 3 o'clock hour to stop whatever he was doing and pray. He often visited a church or chapel to commune with the Lord. As we conversed about the importance of this practice, he reminded me of Jesus' words to St. Faustina.

I remind you, My daughter, that as often as you hear the clock strike the third hour, immerse yourself completely in My mercy, adoring and glorifying it; invoke its omnipotence for the whole world, and particularly for poor sinners; for at that moment mercy was opened wide for every soul. In this hour you can obtain everything for yourself and for others for the asking; it was the hour of grace for the whole world — mercy triumphed over justice.

My daughter, try your best to make the Stations of the Cross in this hour; provided that your duties permit it; and if you are not able to make the Stations of the Cross, then at least step into the chapel for a moment and adore, in the Blessed Sacrament, My Heart, which is full of mercy; and should you be unable to step into the chapel, immerse

yourself in prayer there where you happen to be, if only for a brief instant. I claim veneration for My mercy from every creature (*Diary*, 1572).

Reginald tried to pray the Stations of the Cross regularly. He told me that sometimes he would offer this prayer along with the Sorrowful Mysteries of the Rosary. By reflecting on how our Lord suffered for the sake of humanity, Reginald's love for Christ increased each day. He found his time of prayer at the Hour of Great Mercy to be an integral part of his life. It helped bring about the conversion of his heart. Reginald also found himself making various sacrifices to the Lord during this time. For instance, he tried to avoid eating or drinking. He also routinely avoided watching television, listening to the radio, or pursuing other personal pleasures.

In general, Reginald tried to make this time of prayer something private, when he could intimately encounter God without making others aware. However, he still was willing to share the purpose of his 3 o'clock prayer with others. Those with cancer may likewise receive immense healing, strength, and guidance from the Lord by taking time each day to be with Him at this holy hour.

CHAPTER FIVE

Blessed Virgin Mary, Mother of Mercy

Our Lord Jesus gave us His Most Blessed Mother to be our mother. As He was dying on the cross, He said, "Woman, behold, your son" and then to His disciple, "Behold, your mother" (Jn 19:26-27). Many cancer patients have had a special devotion to Our Most Blessed Mother, the Virgin Mary.

As such, they may clearly listen to the words that she spoke to the children at Fatima, "Tell everybody that God gives graces through the Immaculate Heart of Mary. Tell them to ask graces from her, and that the Heart of Jesus wishes to be venerated together with the Immaculate Heart of Mary. Ask them to plead for peace from the Immaculate Heart of Mary, for the Lord has confided the peace of the world to her." (*Our Lady of Fatima's "Peace Plan from Heaven"*; Catholic Treasures, 1950, p. 13).

Our Lady also implored St. Faustina and her fellow sisters, *Your lives must be like mine: quiet and hidden, in unceasing union with God, pleading for humanity and preparing the world for the second coming of God* (*Diary*, 625).

As St. Faustina and many other saints had a close relationship with Holy Mary, the Mother of God, so must we all. Mother Mary brings us close to her Son, Jesus our Lord. Sue was a woman with a blood cancer who had been hospitalized for a considerable amount of time due to infection and difficulty breathing. Day by day, she received many antibiotics and other measures to support her life. In particular, Sue required oxygen and other treatments to ease her breathing. The life-sustaining therapies she received may have seemed routine to the medical staff caring for her. However, to patients like Sue, such treatment is extraordinary, for it keeps them alive each day.

Sue did not take this for granted, but she was keenly aware that her life was completely in God's hands. He alone was the reason she remained alive. She also understood the importance of the Virgin Mary's intercession as the Mother of God. Mary cared for Jesus and loved Him above all else as both her Son and God. She also loves each of us as her children. As I entered Sue's room each day, her rosary was always out as a wonderful sign of her devotion to Our Blessed Mother. Through Mary, all may receive the tremendous graces that her Son had entrusted her to distribute.

Patients like Sue, devoted to Our Blessed Mother and to praying the Holy Rosary, also help honor her requests that she made to the children at Fatima. The Blessed Mother told the children to sacrifice themselves for sinners. While they performed sacrifices, the children followed Mary's instructions to pray, "O my Jesus, I offer this for love of Thee, for the conversion of poor sinners, and in reparation for all the sins committed against the Immaculate Heart of Mary." (*Our Lady of Fatima's "Peace Plan from Heaven,"* p.6)

As I spent time in oncology, I had the pleasure to work with Reggie. This man had a deep devotion to Mary. Reggie recognized that Mary as Jesus' mother was the surest way to God. Mary humbly acknowledged that it was God who accomplished all the good in her life. As Reggie and I conversed, I learned of his reflection on the Magnificat of the Blessed Mother. He found this prayer to be a wonderful way to praise Almighty God. Mary's Magnificat was proclaimed in great humility, acknowledging the justice of God but also honoring His great mercy.

Mary said, "My soul proclaims the greatness of the Lord; my spirit rejoices in God my savior. For He has looked upon His handmaid's lowliness; behold, from now on will all ages call me blessed. The Mighty One has done great things for me, and holy is His name. His mercy is from age to age to those who fear Him. He has shown might with His arm, dispersed the arrogant of mind and heart. He has thrown down the rulers from their thrones but lifted up the lowly.

The hungry He has filled with good things; the rich He has sent away empty. He has helped Israel His servant, remembering His mercy, according to His promise to our fathers, to Abraham and to his descendants forever" (Lk 1:46-55).

Reggie learned from this great prayer that we, like Mary, must acknowledge that by ourselves we are nothing. Yet by coming to the Lord in great humility, we allow Him to do wonderful things in our lives. Reggie had come from a middle-class family, and he said he had taken many things for granted as he grew up. Whether it be the food he ate, the clothes he wore, the schools he attended, or even the family of which he was a part, Reggie assumed he was entitled to all these things.

However, as he aged and experienced various losses in life, his heart gradually changed. As he began to spend time with cancer patients, he encountered many holy souls. These patients and families taught him to cherish everything in life. Reggie began to deeply appreciate his morning bagel, his glass of water at lunch, and the time he had with his wife and son, which were all wonderful gifts from God. The Blessed Mother helped transform his life. Reggie then also came to sing, "My soul proclaims the greatness of the Lord; my spirit rejoices in God my savior."

Cancer patients can receive great strength from praying to Mary and invoking her intercession. A wonderful devotion to honor the Virgin Mary is to recall her Seven Sorrows, of which she informed St. Bridget. These include the prophecy of holy Simeon, who predicted how she and her Son would suffer. Some patients' families suffer terribly at the news their loved ones have cancer and will eventually die from this disease.

The next sorrow was Our Blessed Mother's flight into Egypt with the Child Jesus and St. Joseph, when King Herod sought to destroy the Christ Child. Those with cancer may feel the threat of death and run for help. This sometimes is accomplished by seeking medical attention, but more importantly, such souls may take flight and find true refuge in Mary and our Lord Jesus Christ.

Mary's third sorrow was the loss of the Child Jesus in the Temple. Some families whose loved ones face cancer also experience great loss. This may result from patients requiring much time in the hospital and being removed from their normal family lives. In other cases, those with cancer may become withdrawn, perhaps due to depression or ultimately from dying.

The fourth sorrow occurred when Jesus met Mary on the way of the cross. Judy was a mother who wept with deep sorrow as her son was dying from multiple organ failure after having his cancer treated. As I looked in her eyes filled with tears, it was clear she shared every bit of her son's suffering. This gave me a brief glimpse of what Mary must have felt as she embraced Jesus on His way of the cross.

The fifth sorrow she experienced was Jesus' crucifixion. As patients die in oncology, they are often surrounded by loved ones. In such cases, prayers are commonly said for those loved ones who are dying, and silence may speak volumes. Everything else in their lives is placed aside while they focus completely on their loved ones who face death.

The sixth sorrow of Our Blessed Mother was the taking down of Jesus' Body from the cross after His death. Louise was the wife of Sam, who was another cancer patient of mine. She had provided Sam constant support during his treatment. Louise displayed strong courage as her husband was dying. However, it was not until after his death that Louise broke down in sorrow. Like many other caregivers of cancer patients, she had tremendous resolve as she helped carry her loved one's cross.

The seventh sorrow of Our Blessed Mother was the burial of Jesus. Although the burial act is the final physical separation a person has with a departed loved one, it provides an opportunity for intercessory prayer, which may be offered for deceased patients and their families.

The Blessed Mother informed St. Bridget of seven graces that would be granted to souls who honor her daily by saying seven Hail Marys and meditating on her sorrows. Such a practice provides strength and grace to cancer patients and their loved ones. The first grace is granting peace to their families. Second is enlightenment about the divine mysteries. Third,

Mary said that she will console them in their pains, and she will accompany them in their work.

Fourth, Our Lady informs us she will give them as much as they ask for, as long as it does not oppose "the adorable will" of Jesus or the sanctification of their souls. Fifth, the Virgin Mary tells us she will defend them in their spiritual battles with the infernal enemy and that she will protect them at every instant of their lives. Sixth, she lets us know she will visibly help them at the moment of their death and that they will see the face of their mother. Finally, Our Blessed Mother states that those who propagate this devotion to her sorrows will be taken directly from earthly life to eternal happiness, since all their sins will be forgiven, and she and Jesus will be their eternal consolation and joy.

Father Ed was an older priest who was a chaplain at a veterans' hospital. As he visited the patients throughout the hospital, he brought the Lord's mercy to many souls. Father Ed found his ministry challenging. Each day, he encountered different patients. Some may have had cancers or other life-threatening illnesses, which would soon take their lives. Father Ed seemed most concerned about those with hardened hearts, who would not turn from their evil ways and repent. God's mercy is a wonderful gift, freely available to all, but we need to be open and willing to receive it. As Fr. Ed recognized this truth, he was firm with those who needed correction. Yet his sincere desire was for souls to repent from sin and return to God.

Amidst these frustrating encounters, Fr. Ed would make time to pray. He loved celebrating Mass, which was the greatest prayer he could offer for souls. Then he would spend time with our Lord in the Most Blessed Sacrament. He also had a strong devotion to Mary. She was clearly his guide to Jesus, and he wished to share his love for Mary with others.

Father Ed taught that when we pray, we should do so for Our Lady's intentions. He stated that in doing so, we know that we are praying for the best of intentions. Our Blessed Mother Mary is closest to God, so with her great love for each of us, she helps us to know His holy will. Father Ed also helped souls to know the importance of loving and honoring the Blessed Mother. In doing so, we imitate Jesus, who loved and honored His holy mother.

From the Holy Scriptures, we learn how God's gift of mercy has also been spread through holy mothers. For instance, in the Second Book of Maccabees, the Israelites were being persecuted by a pagan king. In particular, if the Israelites did not renounce their faith and eat pork in violation of God's law, they were put to death. One remarkable family consisted of a mother with seven sons. She encouraged her children to remain faithful to God, despite the violent persecution they were enduring.

Each son stood up for their faith. In the midst of great darkness, they remained hopeful due to the witness of their mother. She had strengthened their faith and helped give them courage to trust in God. Her sons were tortured as this holy woman watched them be killed, one by one. She acknowledged that her sons were given to her by Almighty God and that He would raise them up at the resurrection (see 2 Macc 7:1-42).

Likewise, Our Blessed Mother watched her innocent Son die a horrible death full of shame and dishonor. Holy Mary remained by her Son's side in good times and bad as He proclaimed the truth and gave Himself to us as the Word of God.

A former patient of mine named Mitch had an extraordinary mother who inspired him. She had just lost her husband, and then Mitch developed acute leukemia. Before she could get over the shock and grief of life without her husband, this mother had to face her son's aggressive cancer. Each day, she remained at Mitch's side. She watched her son endure tremendous suffering.

There were good days on occasion but also plenty of more challenging ones. Mitch developed life-threatening infections, bleeding, nausea, diarrhea, and other problems day by day. Although he was a courageous, young man who tended not to complain, his mother knew well that he was suffering considerably at times. She continually offered Mitch love and support.

Sometimes his mother may have had little to say. However, she would just sit and watch Mitch. In these times of holy silence, their relationship grew further. The important thing that Mitch needed to know each day was that someone was with him through it all. This woman was, therefore, not only his mother, but she was also the one who helped bring Christ into his life. In such trying circumstances, she taught me the importance of not focusing on oneself. As the Blessed Mother had brought Christ to others, Mitch's mom tried to do so as well. This holy woman was a wonderful example for all caretakers as she helped her son embrace and carry his cross until death.

The Blessed Mother instructs us to do whatever her Son tells us just as she spoke to the servants at the wedding feast of Cana (see Jn 2:5). As our loving mother, she truly knows what is best for us. She is merciful and pleads for us to Jesus, invoking His unfathomable mercy. Each of us is called to listen, therefore, to her Son. In particular, we are to feed the hungry, give drink to the thirsty, welcome the stranger, clothe the naked, care for the ill, and visit those in prison (see Mt 25:35-36). Above all, the Blessed Mother shows us how to best listen to her Son by the example of her own life. By the grace of God, she perfectly followed Jesus' commandment, "Love one another as I love you" (Jn 15:12).

CHAPTER SIX

The Holy Rosary

The Holy Rosary is a great gift from Our Lady that is treasured by the Catholic Church, including many cancer patients. Patients who are suffering often have maintained a deep sense of peace due to their devotion to the Rosary. While these individuals are confined to their hospital rooms, they may enter deeply into the mysteries of this great prayer and avoid many of the distractions in life that so many others encounter. In doing so, they may obtain tremendous graces for themselves as well as for others while advancing towards holiness.

Tradition has it that Mary gave the Holy Rosary to St. Dominic as a means to intimately encounter the Lord. The prayer begins by making the "Sign of the Cross" to invoke the Blessed Trinity. Then we pray the Apostles' Creed, from which we declare our faith in the Triune God. It also unifies the Church as we pray for the Communion of Saints. Then healing is prayed for through the forgiveness of sins. Finally, this prayer allows us to express our great hope in the resurrection from the dead and life everlasting.

Before praying the Mysteries, many recite as introductory prayers one "Our Father," three "Hail Marys," and one "Glory Be." Each decade is then dedicated to a specific mystery of Jesus' life or that of the Blessed Virgin Mary. As one begins to contemplate each mystery, we start with the "Our Father," centering our prayers and thoughts on Almighty God. In particular, we pray this invoking God's mercy. With the words, "forgive us our trespasses as we forgive those who trespass against us," we are challenged to be people of mercy as well. By following Jesus and closely imitating His life, we share in the hope of forgiveness for our sins. By being people of mercy, we have nothing to fear, for our actions are then in harmony with those of Christ's life.

Ten "Hail Marys" are prayed, enabling communion with Our Blessed Mother. As we honor her with these prayers, she may perfect them and bring them before Almighty God. A "Glory be" is next offered up to praise the Triune God. We can then conclude each decade with the Fatima Prayer: "O my Jesus, forgive us our sins, save us from the fires of hell, lead all souls to heaven, especially those in most need of Thy mercy."

The Holy Rosary then culminates with the "Hail, Holy Queen," which is prayed to acknowledge our Mother of Mercy. She is our great advocate and guide. At the end of the Holy Rosary, many also pray one "Our Father," "Hail Mary," and "Glory be," offering them for the intentions of our Holy Father as part of a plenary indulgence.

Mary was a woman who was devoted to Our Blessed Mother. She prayed for the Virgin Mary's intercession to bring about healing through Project Mercy. This included praying for life and an end to abortion, for the poor souls in purgatory, and for God's holy will to be done. Instead of going through an extensive list of petitions each day, this prayer places all of one's intentions into Our Blessed Mother's hands. Therefore, as we pray for Project Mercy, our individual prayers not spoken will also be heard. Prayer in this manner redirects the focus from self to God through Mary. God our loving Father knows well what we need before we even have a faint thought of asking for something. By placing God's will first, we transform our lives into that of Jesus' life as He prayed in the Garden of Gethsemane, "Father ... not what I will but what You will" (Mk 14:36).

Mary found that her life was changed, and she helped others to understand the importance of heeding Our Blessed Mother's requests. The focus of her prayer was on God's mercy for all. This was in perfect harmony with that of Jesus' Gospel message, the teachings of the Church, and the message of Our Blessed Mother at Fatima.

Mary's efforts helped bring others closer to the Lord. Many people came and prayed with her, including those with various infirmities. People came together to seek further healing in their lives. In particular, Mary's prayer groups fervently prayed the Holy Rosary to intercede for sinners. Before all the Holy Masses at her parish, the Rosary was prayed. It was wonderful to see. In some circumstances, though, Mary faced criticism. Yet she and her fellow parishioners were persistent in honoring the Blessed Mother's request. They were not ashamed to follow the call to pray the Holy Rosary for the world's healing.

The Joyful Mysteries

In the Joyful Mysteries, those with cancer may find a refreshed spirit as they share in the lives of Our Blessed Mother and the Child Jesus. The Archangel Gabriel's Annunciation to Mary that she was to be the Mother of the Savior initially may have troubled her. However, without hesitation, she said "yes" to God and became an integral part of the salvation of mankind (see Lk 1:26-38). Likewise, patients with cancer are often faced with many uncertainties, but in saying "yes" to God's will, they can offer their sufferings for the good of humanity. This allows them to also imitate Our Blessed Mother Mary, who declared she was the handmaid of the Lord.

In the Visitation, the second Joyful Mystery, we hear how the Virgin Mary was concerned not with her own condition, but instead she went in haste to the hill country to help her elderly cousin, St. Elizabeth (see Lk 1:39-45). Frequently, patients with cancer also do not merely worry about how their illness is affecting their own lives. Rather, they may show concern for their families, who are trying to carry on without them being able to function in their normal capacity. In this love for others, despite their own hardships, these individuals bring Jesus to others as Our Blessed Mother brought Christ to St. Elizabeth's home. We should welcome such patients into our lives as St. Elizabeth welcomed the Virgin Mary and Jesus into her life.

From the Nativity, the third Joyful Mystery, we see the profound humility of Jesus as He took the form of a helpless infant (see Lk 2:8-14). Many cancer patients experience a regression from a state of normal health to one of complete dependence on others. However, as they reflect on the great love and mercy of God in the Incarnation of our Lord Jesus, they may come to more closely imitate Christ by placing their lives into God's hands.

As patients contemplate this mystery of the Rosary, they may also experience Our Blessed Mother and St. Joseph bringing Jesus to them. Even though the infant Jesus may have seemed insignificant to the world, the lowly shepherds came to know of His glory. The angels appeared to them, proclaiming, "Glory to God in the highest and on earth peace to those on whom His favor rests" (Lk 2:14).

Likewise, as those with cancer humble themselves, they become more prepared to receive Jesus into their lives. For instance, those who are in the hospital on Christmas do not have parties to attend, trees to decorate, gifts to wrap, or other rushing about that many others seem so focused on during the Advent and Christmas season. It is during this time that they may establish an intimate relationship with their Savior.

Not only can these patients be the recipients of profound grace, they also may be the instruments that God uses to touch others' lives. By attaining lives of exemplary holiness, these individuals may act like the angels who announced Christ Jesus' birth to the shepherds. Some cancer patients have needed to be hospitalized for weeks or months during this time of the year.

As I have visited such patients, I have experienced the presence of Jesus Christ, as if I had walked into the stable in Bethlehem where He was born over 2,000 years ago. In these patients' hearts resides our merciful Savior who is waiting for us to come to Him. I find it sad that some patients remain confined in the hospital for long periods of time without ever having any family or friends come to visit.

Just as Jesus is distraught about lukewarm souls and those who refuse to come to Him, these patients who remain in solitude may experience a similar sorrow. These individuals are often the instruments of mercy that our Lord uses to pour out graces upon souls. Jesus tells us that He will reward those who came to Him when He was sick or in prison. Then the just will ask "Lord ... when did we see You ill or in prison, and visit You?" He will answer them, "... whatever you did for one of these least brothers of Mine, you did for Me" (Mt 25:37-40).

The mystery of the Lord's Presentation in the Temple, the fourth Joyful Mystery, reveals to us the importance of coming to God's sanctuary where we may encounter Him intimately (see Lk 2:22-38). Although ideally this occurs during our celebration of Holy Mass and Eucharistic Adoration, we can also experience our Lord's holy presence anytime and anyplace. Through the Sacrament of Baptism, one becomes a Temple of the Holy Spirit. Many patients grow in deep holiness by allowing the Lord to come into their souls. At the Presentation of the Christ Child in the Temple, we hear how Our Blessed Mother and St. Joseph made an offering of turtledoves to the Lord. A number of my patients continually pray and offer up their sufferings to God as a similar holy sacrifice.

Simeon and Anna were elderly individuals who through the grace of the Holy Spirit came to recognize the Child Jesus as the Savior of the world. Likewise, often cancer patients have a similar deep faith in Jesus Christ. The Gospel message becomes such a wonderful way of life for them that they want to share it with everyone they encounter. Sadly, others around them may not accept or cherish such a deep faith in Jesus, as likely some who had heard Simeon and Anna neglected to accept Jesus. Yet many who hear the Word of God and see it alive in such individuals do change their lives. Hence, the kingdom of God continues to grow in our midst.

In the fifth Joyful Mystery of the Finding of the Christ Child in the Temple, the importance of communing with Almighty God in His Holy dwelling place is further pondered. Although St. Joseph and the Blessed Mother searched through-out Jerusalem for three days before they found Jesus, it was only when they came to the Temple that they attained the One whom their hearts so greatly desired (see Lk 2:41-52).

When I think of this mystery, I remember being at my parish church for a series of evening talks by a visiting priest during Lent. The week ended with Holy Mass, Eucharistic Adoration, and a long procession of the Most Blessed Sacrament throughout the church. The priest kept stopping for people to venerate and touch the base of the monstrance.

As I observed the many people communing with our Lord, I noticed one woman reach through the crowd to touch the monstrance. I then recognized Kathleen, a patient of mine with relapsed acute leukemia. Despite her severe illness, from which she shortly thereafter died, she made her way through the winter weather to my church for this special encounter with our Lord Jesus. The immense love she had for Christ as she sought Him in the Mass and the Most Blessed Sacrament was a powerful witness of the need to continually search for God despite all obstacles in life.

The Luminous Mysteries

Our Lord's Baptism is the first Luminous Mystery of the Rosary. As we reflect on Jesus' submission during this holy event, we hear our heavenly Father say, "This is My beloved Son, with whom I am well pleased" (Mt 3:17). Some cancer patients may never have been baptized and, therefore, seek this great Sacrament during their illness. However, others may use their time of sickness to renew their Baptismal promises. As Christ's Baptism was the initiating event that began His public life, this holy Sacrament brings all who receive it to a new life regardless of their state of physical health.

I helped care for one hospitalized cancer patient named Tim, who strongly desired Baptism by submersion under water before he died. Unfortunately, his hospital room had no tub, and he was attached to a number of intravenous lines and catheters that made his wish seem impossible to carry out. One of the physician assistants on the medical ward, however, found out that a whirlpool was available in another part of the hospital. Tim was able to make his way to this pool for Baptism, and shortly thereafter, he died. Through such acts,

I remain in awe at how Almighty God works through His children to pour out His mercy.

In the second Luminous Mystery, we hear of Jesus' self-manifestation at the wedding feast of Cana (see Jn 2:1-11). We reflect on how Jesus performed His first public miracle at the request of His Immaculate Mother. Many cancer patients have a special devotion to Our Blessed Mother. When Mary told Jesus about the wedding couple's need at Cana, it was certain He would meet those needs. So, too, does she promptly assist all who entrust her with their concerns.

This mystery of the Rosary also teaches us how Jesus uses the servants' obedience to help complete the miracle. As we learn to obey our Lord's commands, we, too, may assist Almighty God in His miraculous work here on earth. We also see in this mystery the transformation of water into wine, which prefigured our Lord's transubstantiation of water and wine into His Most precious Blood in the Holy Eucharist.

Jesus also used this event to elevate Matrimony to the dignity of a sacrament. Many patients and their spouses have been exemplary models of true Christian marriage. I have witnessed innumerable cancer patients whose faithful spouses supported them throughout their illnesses. In doing so, they brought Jesus to their loved ones. This holy union between husband and wife has thus often been compared with the loving relationship of Jesus Christ and His Church.

In the third Luminous Mystery, we hear of Jesus' proclamation of the kingdom of God as He calls us all to conversion. Jesus tells us that He came to call sinners and not the righteous. We are also told to love the Lord our God with all of our hearts, minds, bodies, souls, and strength, and to love our neighbors as ourselves. This mystery also brings to light the Beatitudes (see Mt 5:3-12).

As we hear "Blessed are the poor in spirit, for theirs is the kingdom of heaven" (Mt 5:3), I recall the many humble souls who have struggled with their cancers. Their suffering brought them glory in the eyes of Almighty God. "Blessed are they who mourn, for they will be comforted" (Mt 5:4) may bring solace to those individuals who are distraught about their diseases. "Blessed are the meek, for they shall inherit the land" (Mt 5:5) is the beatitude that rewards the humble souls. Many patients with cancer come to master this virtue, and it is to such as these that our Lord gives the new world of His kingdom.

Then we read, "Blessed are they who hunger and thirst for righteousness, for they will be satisfied" (Mt 5:6). Despite many patients' desires to prolong their earthly lives and to increase their material possessions, those who have detached themselves from the things of this world to focus their lives on God will not go unrewarded.

Those who treasure The Divine Mercy message and devotion rejoice as we hear our Lord next say, "Blessed are the merciful, for they will be shown mercy" (Mt 5:7). This great gift of forgiveness allows many suffering souls to receive true healing for themselves and others. "Blessed are the clean of heart, for they will see God" (Mt 5:8). Some with cancer develop a sincerity of heart, which allows them to love. Their lack of duplicity in dealing with others enables them to encounter the Lord.

Such patients may also be true examples of peace to the world, reflecting the verse, "Blessed are the peacemakers, for they will be called children of God" (Mt 5:9). Our Lord then concludes by telling us "Blessed are they who are persecuted for the sake of righteousness, for theirs is the kingdom of heaven. Blessed are you when they insult you and persecute you and utter every kind of evil against you because of Me. Rejoice and be glad, for your reward will be great in heaven" (Mt 5:10-12). Despite facing potentially life-threatening diseases, many of those with cancer find that such persecutions and insults are far worse things to suffer. Yet, rather than despairing, these individuals should be consoled by our Lord Jesus' Word that never loses its force or power to heal.

In the fourth Luminous Mystery of our Lord's Transfiguration, we see the glory of Jesus revealed to His disciples (see Mt 17:1-8). Joan was a woman with relapsed acute leukemia after a bone marrow transplant. She helped me better appreciate this mystery by her example. As Jesus was transfigured to strengthen His Apostles' faith in Him before His Passion and death, Joan fortified those who were distraught about her illness.

Although she faced death, Joan radiated great joy, peace, and love upon her family and friends. Saint Peter asked our Lord if he should make three tents, one for Jesus, one for Moses, and another for Elijah. However, from a cloud that overshadowed them came the voice of the Father: "This is My beloved Son, with whom I am well pleased; listen to Him" (Mt 17:5). In a similar manner, Joan had others come to honor her before her death. Yet being a woman of great faith, I believe that she, too, would have preferred others to listen to our Lord and trust in His mercy and love rather than to express needless worry about her welfare. Jesus' glorious splendor shines continually on the world through such humble and loving souls.

As the three Apostles were lying in fear on the ground after hearing the voice from the cloud, Jesus told them, "Rise, and do not be afraid" (Mt 17:7). He continues to speak these same words to each of us, no matter what fears in life we may face.

The fifth Luminous Mystery is our Lord's institution of the Holy Eucharist at the Last Supper (see Mt 26:26-29). Here we recall our Lord's awesome gift of Himself as He promised to remain with us until the end of time. This Sacrament is a gift beyond all comprehension, and we can only accept it with faith from Almighty God. Innumerable souls have benefited from the graces outpoured from reception of the Holy Eucharist. Although many cancer patients benefit from medical treatments while others do not, all may receive healing through the Holy Eucharist.

During my medical training, I encountered a man with cancer. His name was Sam. He was critically ill, in the intensive care unit on extensive life support measures. His family was aware of his critical condition, and they sought for him to receive the Most Holy Eucharist. Though Sam was unable to swallow a complete host, they requested that only a small portion, the size of a crumb, be given.

Their great faith reminded me of that displayed by the woman in the Gospel who had a hemorrhage for 12 years (see Mk 5:25-34). She was unable to be helped by any doctor. Yet as she approached Jesus, she said, "If I but touch his clothes, I shall be cured." By receiving just a minute portion of the Eucharist, Sam's family also knew that their loved one would receive healing, as he was able to commune with God. The Most Holy Eucharist is a great gift that has brought about physical healings for many patients. However, far more importantly, it brings about spiritual healings for all who receive God with faith.

The Sorrowful Mysteries

As we enter the Sorrowful Mysteries of the Rosary, we first reflect on our Lord's agony in the Garden of Gethsemane (see Lk 22:39-46). At that time, Jesus knew well what awaited Him as He entered into His Passion. Every physical blow, cruel remark, personal betrayal, and rejection taunted our Lord in the Garden. He told St. Faustina that lukewarm souls caused His soul the most dreadful loathing in the Garden of Olives. They were the reason He cried out, **"Father, take this cup away from Me, if it be Your will"** (*Diary*, 1228). Jesus further spoke of such souls to St. Faustina, saying, **All the graces that I pour out upon them flow off them as off the face of a rock** (*Diary*, 1702).

Many with cancer who face suffering and death may be comforted to know that our Lord Jesus was also tempted to run from His Passion and death. However, as our God and perfect role model, Jesus shows us how to embrace suffering for the reparation of sin and the glory of the Lord. It is in these moments of deep suffering, whether physical, emotional, psychological, or spiritual, that God is closest to His children.

Saint Faustina describes such a soul in her *Diary*, saying, "... that during these spiritual torments it is close to God, but it is blind. ... How grave is the malady of the eyes of the soul which, struck by divine light, claims that there is no light, whereas, it is so intense that it blinds her. ... God is closer to a soul at such moments than at others, because it would not be able to endure these trials with the help of ordinary grace alone" (109).

As I reflect on this first Sorrowful Mystery, I also recall Ralph, who had a blood cancer called multiple myeloma (see Glossary). His disease had relapsed after he received many different treatments. When I saw him at an outpatient appointment, he was distraught. Yet Ralph emphatically proclaimed that as a Christian he trusted in the Lord. He firmly believed that even though he would likely die soon, God would take care of his wife and children. He kept saying, "I got to believe that. I got to believe that," as tears poured from his eyes. My heart was deeply saddened by Ralph's great sorrow. However, I also marveled at his trust in the Lord with great admiration. Ralph was a living witness of the suffering face of Christ.

In the second Sorrowful Mystery of the Rosary, we contemplate Jesus' scourging at the pillar (see Mt 27:26). It is horrifying to think that our sweet Lord willingly and full of love underwent this torture for our sins. It is also astonishing that we who, in fact, deserved this punishment inflicted it upon Christ by our sinfulness. Even today, Jesus experiences further scourging when His children are afflicted by others' hatred.

It is discouraging to see cancer patients, who are already suffering, undergo further stress and affliction by others' unkind words and neglect as well as from their lack of understanding, patience, and love. For instance, Jim was a man I had treated for an aggressive lymphoma. He achieved a complete remission, recovered well, and was cured years later. However, as Jim completed his therapy, his wife divorced him.

As I followed Jim over the years, I was always impressed with his profound humility. He never complained during his intense chemotherapy, despite the significant side effects that he experienced. Though he had faced death throughout the time of his treatment, he had shown no fear. However, the rejection by his wife, whom he loved, was a far greater suffering for him. As many patients like Jim endure these and other torments, one can get a small glimpse of what our Lord had suffered during His scourging at the pillar.

The third Sorrowful Mystery is Jesus' crowning with thorns. Here, we see our Lord being humiliated as the crown of thorns is forced into His skull. A reed that was meant to be His "scepter" was used to strike His blessed head, and a purple garment was placed on Him to mock His kingship (see Mk 15:16-20). When we say that Jesus is our King but then sin, we ridicule Him in the same way as the Roman soldiers.

Although cancer patients do not experience the severe humiliation that Jesus endured, they may still feel a lack of respect. As they become dependent on others for basic care needs, some feel a loss of dignity. Even worse, some have considered euthanasia. This evil denies the God-given sanctity of their lives.

Our Lord displayed tremendous courage in this third mystery, and many patients with these deadly diseases seek to follow His example. This includes those with cancer involving the brain, who may have horrible headaches. Through contemplation of this mystery, they may glorify God by offering up their suffering in union with the pain Jesus experienced from the crown of thorns.

We next reflect in the fourth Sorrowful Mystery on Christ carrying His cross to Calvary (see Jn 19:16-17). Not only was our Lord condemned to death, but He was forced to carry His own instrument of destruction. Amidst the hatred and horror He experienced along the *Via Dolorosa*, Jesus met His Blessed Mother. Although His Sacred Heart was likely crushed to see her suffering for Him, Jesus undoubtedly saw her as a light shining in the darkness of that hour. Patients facing death imminently, as well as everyone else who carries the cross with them, can likewise see this light from Mary when we turn to her with love and trust.

John was a patient of mine. He was critically ill in the medical intensive care unit after treatment for his cancer. He had failure of multiple organs and was expected to die quickly.

However, his wife, who was not Catholic, brought in a large picture of Our Blessed Mother that someone from his church had given to her. I recall seeing the picture placed off to the side of his bed, looking over him as he was maintained on a ventilator and other life-support measures.

As the next few weeks passed, John gradually improved, and he was later taken off the ventilator. He was discharged from the hospital and returned to his family at home. This is just one of many examples how Our Lady intercedes for her children as they carry their crosses.

During our trials in life, we need to follow in our Lord's footsteps through the narrow door. This leads to death of the body but then to everlasting life. Along the way, God also places Veronicas, Simons, and others to help us as we carry our crosses. Most importantly, though, Jesus is with us every step of the way. He intercedes for us to the Father. "Because He Himself was tested through what He suffered, He is able to help those who are being tested" (Heb 2:18). ... Son though He was, He learned obedience from what He suffered; and when He was made perfect, He became the source of eternal salvation for all who obey Him ..." (Heb 5:8-9).

In the final Sorrowful Mystery, we contemplate Jesus' death on the cross (see Mt 27:45-52). What a horrifying thought that we all could be such sinners as to kill our God. At the same time, though, we cannot even fathom what a tremendous act of love our Lord performed for each and every one of us through His death at Calvary.

Jesus told St. Faustina, **Pure love gives the soul strength at the very moment of dying. When I was dying on the cross, I was not thinking about Myself, but about poor sinners, and I prayed for them to My Father. I want your last moments to be completely similar to Mine on the cross. There is but one price at which souls are bought, and that is suffering united to My suffering on the cross. Pure love understands these words; carnal love will never understand them** (*Diary*, 324).

Many people die from cancer every day. However, those who embrace their crosses as Jesus did are living witnesses of Christ in our midst. Linda was one such individual. She had fought her chronic leukemia for many years and had received all of the standard therapies for her disease, followed by three bone marrow transplants. After years of fighting, she laid in her hospital bed with her family around her.

She asked me if it was okay to stop treatment and just allow her death to occur. I assured her that this was definitely acceptable, and she later passed quickly from this life. Her resilience during her earthly existence came from her faith in God and her great love for Him and others. Linda imitated Jesus by courageously embracing her sufferings as her earthly life came to its end. By seeing her family around her and knowing that she had fought the good fight, she could follow our Lord's example as He declared, "Father, into Your hands I commend My Spirit." (Lk 23:46). "It is finished" (Jn 19:30). Then He bowed His head and died.

The Glorious Mysteries

In the Glorious Mysteries, we first recall Christ's Resurrection from the dead. We hear of the women going to the tomb on Easter morning. Later, St. Peter and St. John followed (see Jn 20:1-10). As the disciples ardently sought the Lord, so we are called to do the same. We hear that those who first encountered Jesus after His Resurrection did not recognize Him. Mary Magdalene initially wondered whether He was the gardener. The two disciples on the road to Emmaus also did not know Him until the breaking of the bread. Later, the disciples who were fishing at the Sea of Tiberius failed to recognize Him as their resurrected Lord and God.

At first, some cancer patients may not recognize Jesus in their midst. However, as they look closer and search more diligently, they find Him in the many souls who come into their lives. These include family, friends, nurses, doctors, other healthcare workers, and pastoral care ministers. People of faith such as these patients should rejoice, for Jesus told St.

Thomas, "Blessed are those who have not seen and have believed" (Jn 20:29).

When we think of the second Glorious Mystery of our Lord's Ascension into heaven, we remember how He first instructed His disciples, saying, "All power in heaven and on earth has been given to Me. Go, therefore, and make disciples of all nations, baptizing them in the name of the Father, and of the Son, and of the Holy Spirit, teaching them to observe all that I have commanded you. And behold, I am with you always, until the end of the age" (Mt 28:18-20). These words of Christ entrust us with a charge to evangelize the world. It is amazing how many cancer patients, despite their sufferings, can often effectively carry out this holy work. In doing so, they honor God as the Apostles did by falling down and giving Jesus homage as He ascended into heaven.

With the third Glorious Mystery, the Descent of the Holy Spirit upon the disciples and the Blessed Mother at the first Pentecost, we recall the birthday of the Church (see Acts 2:1-4). The Holy Spirit stirs into flame Christ's Church for its mission to evangelize the world.

George was a patient with brain cancer that gradually resulted in a loss of his ability to think clearly. In addition, he experienced headaches and an inability to care for himself. His wife, Ruth, was devoted to him and tried to remain patient as George lost more and more of his mental capacity. As he suffered physically and emotionally from his condition, others continually prayed for him. In particular, the Holy Rosary was offered up for George in union with the Holy Mass. Such prayers were undoubtedly instrumental in allowing the Holy Spirit to strengthen George on his journey to new life.

The fourth Glorious Mystery is the Assumption of Our Blessed Mother into Heaven. Here we contemplate Holy Mary's reunion with her Son, the Father, and the Holy Spirit, along with the angels and saints.

Cancer patients facing death need also to look to the things above. Their focus must be on Almighty God and His mercy, which will afford them the grace of a happy death and everlasting life. Jacqueline was an older woman with a blood cancer that continued to relapse and progress. Eventually, this cancer resulted in her death.

During the last several months of Jacqueline's life, she continued to struggle daily. In addition to her physical ailments, she had many uncertainties that caused her to suffer psychologically as well. Others prayed for her, offered her encouragement, and showed support. These acts of love, plus requests for Our Blessed Mother's intercession through the Holy Rosary, brought Jacqueline comfort. As she died, I felt she came to peace as her soul was called back to the Lord God.

The final Glorious Mystery is the Coronation of Our Blessed Mother as Queen of Heaven and Earth. This reflection allows us to meditate on Mary's holy role as a powerful Mediatrix, one who channels the Lord's graces to all humanity. Through her intercession as our Queen, we may find favor with Almighty God.

Many cancer patients have faithfully maintained a close relationship with Our Lady as they have daily prayed her Holy Rosary. Without question, the Blessed Mother brings her Divine Son to all such souls who welcome Him and her into their hearts.

PART THREE

Growing in Virtue While Struggling with Cancer

CHAPTER ONE

Humility

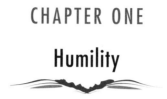

The Lord desires our humble trust in Him, and many cancer patients are living examples of such docility. In the Gospel, we hear that Jesus was invited to a banquet, where He noted how people kept trying to take the seats of honor. Christ tells us that if we take the highest seat and a more distinguished guest arrives, the host may tell us to give up our seat and shamefully go to the lowest seat. Therefore, Jesus advises us to choose the lowest place first, then when the host sees us, he will ask us to move up to a higher position. We will then win the esteem of our fellow guests (see Lk 14:7-11).

Often times in medicine as in other walks of life, those who assert themselves or who are considered powerful attract the most attention and in many cases receive various positions of leadership. However, we hear from Jesus that it is the humble who will be exalted. Those who empty themselves realize that any and all good they do is accomplished through the grace of Almighty God and His mercy. Throughout history and the Bible, we have wonderful examples of those through whom such testimony is given. We hear how Moses was a man of profound humility, and so was King David, who began as a young shepherd. Later, in the New Testament, John the Baptist provided a wonderful model of meekness.

Our Blessed Mother and Almighty God Himself in the person of our Lord Jesus Christ define perfect humility. In the Beatitudes, we hear, "Blessed are the meek, for they will inherit the land" (Mt 5:5). Some cancer patients may have low self-esteem, since their diseases are potentially life threat-ening. However, when one accepts his or her cross, anxiety and fear can significantly decrease or completely disappear.

When patients place their lives in the hands of their physicians, they also practice the virtue of humility. As their relationships with their caregivers further develop, this process often becomes easier. I believe that true compassion and love expressed by healthcare workers allows for the formation of strong relationships with patients. This, in turn, may enable them to cope far better with their illnesses. Likewise, as we completely trust in the unfathomable love and mercy that God has for us all, it becomes natural to humbly submit our lives to His divine will.

Obedience to Almighty God is humility that expresses deep love. When we sincerely love someone, any sacrifice we endure for them is gladly accepted. I have witnessed many cancer patients suffer. Those who offer up their mortifications for the glory of God are wonderful examples for us all. Their lives are a reflection of Jesus, who is the model of perfect humility. The meekness with which the Virgin Mary lived should also strengthen each of us and teach us to follow her magnificent example of trust in Jesus.

Some people may have enjoyed lives of wealth, power, and considerable success in this world that can lead to a feeling of superiority. However, when faced with a cancer, such souls are forced to reexamine their lives. Illness can be the spark to ignite a great spiritual transformation through which they see the world in a new light. The standards by which the world judges are then seen as worthless. Pomp and great success in this world are not the standards by which God judges success. The Lord tells us what He requires of us through the Prophet Micah: "Only to do the right and to love goodness, and to walk humbly with your God" (Mic 6:8).

Jesus is also clear in the Gospel that those who exalt themselves will be humbled, while those who humble themselves will be exalted (see Mt 23:12). He tells us that some who are first will be last, while others who are last will be first. He who is God humbled Himself to become man. Born in abject poverty, He was later rejected, persecuted, and condemned to die a shameful death on the cross. How much more should each of us humble ourselves, since we are nothing without God? As we contemplate the humility of Jesus, our lives should proclaim, "All praise and adoration be Yours, Almighty God!"

Stewart was a famous surgeon who, after his retirement, developed a blood cancer. As he underwent treatment, many physicians helped care for him. Some were considerably younger, including many who were still receiving their medical training.

Stewart told one of the hematology/oncology fellows the following story. There had been a man who was traveling down a large river. Unfortunately, the small boat he had been in turned over amidst the rough waves, and he was thrust out into the torrent. The man was unable to swim due to the strength of the current. He became horrified when he realized that he was rapidly heading towards a great waterfall. As thoughts of imminent death rushed through his mind, he came across a rock protruding from the water. The man grabbed onto part of the rock. This stopped his advance down the river.

A group of adolescents tried to throw the man a rope, but he refused their help, thinking that they were incapable of rescuing him. Later, another older man in a small boat came by to offer assistance. Yet the man in the water feared that this older individual would not be able to pull him into his boat if he were to let go of the rock. Afterwards, a woman with a larger boat came by to try and help. The man declined her offer, since he perceived her to be too weak to actually save him. Shortly thereafter, the man lost his grip, was washed away from the rock, and met his death after going over the waterfall.

Later, he stood before the Lord and asked why God did not rescue him when he cried for help. The Lord then told him that He sent the adolescents, the older man, and the woman, but he would not accept their assistance due to his pride.

Stewart then acknowledged it would likewise be foolish for him to refuse the help that the younger physicians were trying to provide him as he faced his cancer. He felt that the Lord put these people in his life for a reason. Stewart displayed great humility and had deep respect for these people. In this, he challenged people to examine their own lives and remember that the Lord works through others to accomplish His purpose.

Jesus further tells us of His desire for humility in the parable of the two men going to the Temple to pray (see Lk 18:9-14). One was a Pharisee who thanked God for all the good things he had done such as fasting, giving alms, paying tithes, and not being like sinners. The other man was a tax collector who did not even dare raise his eyes to heaven. All he did was pray, "O God, be merciful to me a sinner" (Lk 18:13). Jesus said that this man was justified as he left the Temple but not the Pharisee.

Our Lord teaches us once again that he who exalts himself will be humbled, while he who humbles himself will be exalted. Many cancer patients learn the true meaning of humility by facing their serious illnesses. They often submit to the wills of their caregivers and their families as they empty themselves. Some who are dying become open with others and share the deep secrets of their hearts that their former pride would not allow them to mention.

Larry was a man of such humility. He suffered from a recurrent lymphoma and faced an enormous number of treatments. His treatments included intravenous chemotherapies that lowered his blood counts and caused him to lose his hair. In addition, since the cancer involved his central nervous system, he also required chemotherapy to be injected directly into his spinal fluid. He had a special reservoir placed under his scalp by a neurosurgeon.

Larry responded well, despite the side effects. I recall speaking to a priest who knew him well. He informed me that Larry was amazingly accepting of his illness. He also was a Eucharistic minister and a devout Catholic, who recognized that his strength came from God.

In contrast, Rita was a woman who presented to my outpatient clinic for a follow-up visit before being hospitalized to receive chemotherapy for her cancer. At that time, she felt depressed. When I inquired further what most concerned her, Rita told me it was not the chemotherapy, being away from her family, or suffering. Rather, she found it too difficult to give up her task of managing her family's finances and letting her husband perform this work.

Often, when one is too accustomed to a "normal" pace of life and change occurs, it results in considerable anxiety. However, if one can submit his or her will to that of Almighty God's divine will in a spirit of humility, all things are possible. Our Blessed Mother Mary is the perfect example of submission to God's will. In her Magnificat, we hear how God favors the humble (see Lk 1:52). When I think of patients who accept difficulties, I am humbled. By comparison, so many others, including myself, often complain about minor inconveniences like a common cold.

Most patients with cancer seem to know their own bodies better than anyone else. When they notice a new symptom, they report it to their physician. After healthcare providers review symptoms with patients and perform further evaluations, a diagnosis and treatment plan is usually established. However, some patients' presentations do not fall under a textbook description for a specific illness.

This is particularly true when there are atypical manifestations of a disease. In such cases, it is important for healthcare providers to maintain a sense of humility if they are uncertain of a patient's problem. Often one speaks of thinking "outside the box" in these situations. In particular, when dealing with things of the spirit, we must be open to the Lord's inspiration and guidance, for God knows best. It is often the meek and receptive souls who receive the greatest graces, for they recognize their dependence on Almighty God and His great mercy.

Jesus was not accepted by His own kinsfolk when He returned to Nazareth during His public ministry (see Lk 4:16-30). Similarly, some cancer patients feel rejection as they return to their family and friends with a new outlook centered on God and His infinite mercy. As they try to share this message of mercy, they have to humble themselves and accept rejection. Just as our Master and Savior Jesus Christ had to suffer, all who follow Him must be prepared to face similar difficulties (see Jn 15:18-20).

We hear in the Gospel that Jesus thanked His Father for revealing the mysteries of the kingdom to children and the simple while keeping them hidden from the learned and clever (see Lk 10:21). Jesus also said, "Amen, I say to you, unless you turn and become like children, you will not enter the kingdom of heaven. Whoever humbles himself like this child is the greatest in the kingdom of heaven. And whoever receives one child such as this in My name receives Me" (Mt 18:3-5). As such, this should remind us always to be simple and meek of heart, trusting in the Lord as little children.

Often cancer patients regress during their illnesses, not necessarily from their physical ailments but rather psychologically or emotionally. Things that these individuals used to routinely do such as work, caring for others, or even taking care of themselves may no longer be possible, or at least not in the same capacity in which they were previously accustomed.

In this so-called regression, they may find themselves dependent on others to varying degrees. Above all, many may come to realize their absolute dependence on Almighty God. For some, this may have been the first time in their lives that this has occurred. In such a state, these souls may become like the simple children our Lord refers to in the Gospel. They may change their lives accordingly to be open to the graces and mercy of God.

Saint Paul wrote, "Consider your own calling, brothers. Not many of you were wise by human standards, not many were powerful, not many were of noble birth. Rather, God chose the foolish of the world to shame the wise, and God chose the weak of the world to shame the strong, and God chose the lowly and despised of the world, those who count for nothing, to reduce to nothing those who are something, so that no human being might boast before God. It is due to Him that you are in Christ Jesus, who became for us wisdom from God, as well as righteousness, sanctification, and redemption, so that, as it is written, 'Whoever boasts, should boast in the Lord'" (1 Cor 1:26-31).

Although some with cancer may appear weak in the eyes of the world, God often uses them to pour out His love, mercy, and goodness on others. Their faith in Jesus Christ provides them with wisdom, righteousness, sanctification, and redemption. An old tarnished instrument may appear to be worthless. However, when played by a highly talented musician, beautiful music may resound. How much more beautiful will the music be when the Holy Spirit permeates a receptive and trusting soul that loves God and is open to His divine will. Jesus tells us, "Come to Me, all you who labor and are burdened, and I will give you rest. Take My yoke upon you and learn from Me, for I am meek and humble of heart; and you will find rest for yourselves. For My yoke is easy, and My burden light" (Mt 11:28-30). Cancer patients can be inspired by our Lord's words, which may motivate them to grow in holiness and service to God and others.

During my first year of hematology/oncology training, I had the opportunity to help care for an older man named Frank. He had advanced prostate cancer that had spread widely throughout his bones. Frank's senior physician was an international expert highly respected in the medical community. After he had prescribed a certain treatment, Frank developed persistent nausea.

The physician looked at Frank's overall cancer condition rather than focusing on the nausea, which was the complaint that bothered him most. Although this physician may have meant well with Frank's best interest in mind, Frank did not feel he was being listened to, which lead to discontent. Care must be taken when ministering to the sick to provide the attention that they need. This is important for them not to feel as if they are only a number amidst many other patients.

It became readily apparent to me that the soul of each patient must be approached with a spirit of humility and compassion, no matter how busy one is at any time. As the months went by, my relationship with Frank grew. In many of our encounters, I would listen to him without providing any elegant discussion about treating his cancer. Frank also touched my life greatly, for as he was facing death, he made it clear that I was his doctor. Though there are many different honors and awards that physicians may receive, this humble man's gesture of love and trust in me during my early years of training made a deep impression on me. I treasured his acceptance of me as his physician more than many other rewards one could receive in medicine.

The support, love, and mercy that Frank showed to me were a great source of encouragement. They had helped me to grow further as a physician and as a brother in Christ Jesus to others. Many cancer patients can likewise do great things in a spirit of humility and mercy, even when they are gravely ill.

Some cancer patients who become critically ill may be transferred to a medical intensive care unit, where they may require full medical support to resuscitate them. Ventilators may be employed to support one's breathing, medications may be administered to maintain an adequate blood pressure, and infections can be treated. Numerous tubes and intravenous lines may be placed into patients' bodies to deliver this therapy and to monitor their condition. Such intensive support is likewise required for those near spiritual death.

As a soul is deeply affected by mortal sin, its life fades rapidly, and all available sources of spiritual assistance are required to maintain its existence. Such help comes from others praying for the person, offering sacrifices such as fasting and almsgiving, and most importantly, through the celebration of Holy Mass. The graces from these offerings give the soul in a state of severe spiritual illness the opportunity to become "stabilized" spiritually. However, it is critical for further intervention through the Sacrament of Reconciliation and atonement for one's sins to bring about the definitive healing necessary to return the soul to a state of grace and thus to life. A person must be humble of heart to sincerely repent of sin in order for this healing to occur.

Since Pentecost, the Church has been guided by an outpouring of the Holy Spirit, who vivifies her with His life. Fernando had been ill from a recurrence of his blood cancer, and he spent many weeks in the hospital. He spoke no English, but he was a man of faith. As I saw Fernando daily in the hospital, I often had an interpreter with me in order to communicate with him. However, his expressions of love and gratitude were manifestations of the Holy Spirit working in his life. Though this did not occur through the English language, Fernando's gentle mannerisms, sincere humility, and life of virtue were reflections of the face of Christ shining upon others.

Saint Faustina described such souls by saying, "If there is a truly happy soul upon earth, it can only be a truly humble soul. ... A humble soul does not trust itself, but places all its confidence in God. God defends the humble soul and lets Himself into its secrets, and the soul abides in unsurpassable happiness which no one can comprehend" (*Diary*, 593).

Another aspect of humility is to clearly recognize that our knowledge, understanding, and wisdom from the world are finite. In oncology, this is evident from the fact that there are still many diseases we do not understand well. With the lack of effective treatments for such diseases, the outcomes often remain fatal. As such, there remains the need for continuing medical education and recertification board examinations for oncologists and other healthcare professionals in oncology. This process takes considerable time, effort, and resources, but it is clearly necessary to improve treatments and the level of care for those with cancer.

Spiritual healing also requires much effort on the part of each person for his or her good and that of others. This may be accomplished by first recognizing that we are all sinners. We next must sincerely repent. Then, as one proceeds in a true spirit of humility to the tribunal of the Lord's mercy through the Sacrament of Reconciliation, God's graces may be restored and poured out upon the soul. This then cleanses the soul and allows it to become receptive to grace once again. Subsequently, various acts of reparation can be made by the penitent under the direction of the confessor to atone for the wrong he or she has done. One may then advance in holiness and humbly serve the Lord and others.

Saint Faustina felt she was a miserable wretch as she went before the Most Blessed Sacrament. She then heard the words of our Lord, **My daughter, all your miseries have been consumed in the flame of My love, like a little twig** thrown into a roaring fire. **By humbling yourself in this way, you draw upon yourself and upon other souls an entire sea of My mercy** (*Diary*, 178). Souls with cancer, with such a spirit of meekness, bear strong witness to the Gospel message as they trust in God's mercy.

In oncology, as in other areas of medicine, teamwork is of paramount importance. Such unity may be found from collaboration among physicians involved in research. Rather than working for self-glorification by pursuing one's own research alone, many investigators have made considerable strides in the understanding of diseases and in the development of new therapies by working with others for the good of humankind. Unity with the Catholic Church involves submission of the individual's will to that of the Church's authority. By the power of the Holy Spirit, such efforts have preserved the Catholic Church through many heresies, struggles, and persecutions for over 2,000 years.

Love in a spirit of humility may be difficult for those who are ill with cancer. However, one may pray for help to St. Joseph. He knew well what it meant to suffer, to toil, and to love. Although St. Joseph was the head of the Holy Family's household, he demonstrated tremendous humility by putting the needs of Jesus and Mary above his own.

Saint Faustina heard the words of our Lord during a retreat in which He told her, **I am with you. During this retreat, I will strengthen you in peace and in courage so that your strength will not fail in carrying out My designs. Therefore you will cancel out your will absolutely in this retreat and, instead, My complete will shall be accomplished in you. ...** (she was to say) **From today on, my own will does not exist, ... From today on, I do the will of God everywhere, always, and in everything. ... Be afraid of nothing; love will give you strength and make the realization of this easy** (*Diary*, 372). As patients face illnesses such as cancer, they may be strengthened by these words of our Lord. He reassured us that He is with us, that we are not to fear, and that love will be our strength.

Saint Faustina also tells us that a soul who sincerely wants to advance in perfection must strictly observe the advice given by their spiritual director. She stated, "There is as much holiness as there is dependence" (*Diary*, 377). Such obedience and submission of one's will is a true sign of humility.

Saint Faustina's Mother Directress told her, "Sister, let simplicity and humility be the characteristic traits of your soul. Go through life like a little child, always trusting, always full of simplicity and humility, content with everything, happy in every circumstance. There, where others fear, you will pass calmly along, thanks to this simplicity and humility. ... as waters flow from the mountains down into the valleys, so, too, do God's graces flow only into humble souls" (*Diary*, 55).

When one considers the humility of our Lord Jesus, we are left speechless. Consider these words, "Christ Jesus, who, though He was in the form of God, did not regard equality with God, something to be grasped. Rather, He emptied Himself, taking the form of a slave, coming in human likeness; and found human in appearance, He humbled Himself, becoming obedient to death, even death on a cross. Because of this, God greatly exalted Him and bestowed on Him the name that is above every name, that at the name of Jesus every knee should bend, of those in heaven and on earth and under the earth, and every tongue confess that Jesus Christ is Lord to the glory of God the Father!" (Phil 2:5-11).

Jesus not only humbled Himself by taking the form of a poor infant, but even more, through His Passion, death, and Resurrection, He gives us Himself in the Most Holy Eucharist. As one ponders Christ's profound humility and His unfathomable mercy, we can only proclaim, "Jesus, I trust in You!" Our Lord's unconditional love for us inspires us to love Him in return with our whole hearts, souls, bodies, minds, and strength.

As Christ prayed to His heavenly Father before His sorrowful Passion — "... not My will but Yours be done" (Lk 22:42) — so cancer patients who embrace these words during the difficult circumstances of their own lives may be transformed into Christ among us. For some patients, this occurs by accepting the cancer diagnosis. For others, it is committing wholeheartedly to a course of treatment or surgery. For still others, it is accepting death.

As they leave the things of this world behind, such people may develop a spirit of meekness. They are no longer concerned with themselves, and their lives proclaim the words of St. Paul: "... may I never boast except in the cross of our Lord Jesus Christ ..." (Gal 6:14). Some also recognize the great gift of our Lord in the Most Blessed Sacrament and thus center their lives on Him. In this emptying of oneself and spending time with our Lord, one grows in great holiness.

CHAPTER TWO

Service

Jesus taught us that no servant is greater than his master. We must serve others if we are to be merciful like Christ. Jesus also said, "Whoever wishes to be great among you will be your servant; whoever wishes to be first among you will be the slave of all. For the Son of Man did not come to be served but to serve and to give His life as a ransom for many" (Mk 10:43-45).

Many healthcare workers and volunteers take this call of service to heart as they provide care for those who are sick with cancer. We must pray and strive constantly not to become neglectful of those in need, as Jesus warned us with the parable of the rich man and Lazarus (see Lk 16:19-31). The rich man feasted splendidly every day, while Lazarus was left to starve in great poverty on the street. After their deaths, Lazarus rested in the bosom of Father Abraham, while the rich man was left to suffer in the abode of the dead. The rich man's neglect of the poor determined his eternal fate. Though patients with cancer may be limited in their abilities to function normally at home, at work, or in their communities, they remain precious in God's eyes. They possess immortal souls of infinite value. We should give generously to these souls of our time, effort, and love.

However, the "Lazaruses" in the world of oncology are not always patients with cancer. In some cases, patients themselves may be like the rich man in the parable. When a younger healthcare worker such as a nurse, medical student, or intern tries to reach out and provide care, some cancer patients may simply ignore them or look down upon them with disdain. They may feel that these healthcare workers are too young or insignificant to know anything. Other patients might consider them to be unworthy to help manage their medical care.

Yet our Lord Jesus may wish to work through such humble individuals in healthcare to reach patients who have hardened their hearts. A kind word of appreciation or a simple acknowledgement of these healthcare providers' efforts is a way that patients may avoid neglecting opportunities to serve.

When St. Peter told Jesus that His disciples had given up everything to follow Him, he asked what they could expect in return. Jesus assured him, saying "... there is no one who has given up house or wife or brothers or parents or children for the sake of the kingdom of God who will not receive [back] an overabundant return in this present age and eternal life in the age to come" (Lk 18:29-30).

Many healthcare workers and volunteers make tremendous sacrifices throughout their lives in order to minister to the sick. Due to their heavy work schedules, which demand them to provide constant care for cancer patients, such individuals often miss their own family events and other important things in their lives as they work weekends, holidays, and night shifts.

Their patients are also their brothers and sisters in Christ Jesus. Our Lord tells us, "My mother and my brothers are those who hear the word of God and act on it" (Lk 8:21). By caring for those in need with love, mercy, and sacrifice, we are hearing Jesus' Word and putting it into practice.

Often people may be idle and waste the precious gift of time. Our Lord instructs us about this with His parable of a vineyard owner (see Mt 20:1-16). He went out at dawn and hired workers to go and work in his vineyard after they had agreed upon the wage he offered. The owner later went out at 9 a.m., noon, and mid-afternoon to send more workers to his vineyard. Finally, he went out at about 5 p.m. and found more people. He asked them why they had been standing around idle all day. They responded that no one had hired them. The vineyard owner then sent them to work.

In the evening, the owner had the workers come for their pay, beginning with those hired last, who received a full day's wages. When those who were hired first saw this, they thought that they would get more, but they received the same wages. They complained that they had worked through the heat of the day, while those hired last only worked an hour yet received the same wages. The vineyard owner then asked them, "Did you not agree with me for the usual daily wage? … Am I not free to do as I wish with my own money? Are you envious because I am generous?" (Mt 20:13, 15).

These words of our Lord apply well to us still today, for He continually calls souls throughout life, and different individuals respond to His call at different times. The wages are the same for all, everlasting life with Almighty God. We should, therefore, rejoice in the Lord's generosity while responding to His call.

On the oncology wards, extraordinary Eucharistic ministers circulate through the halls to bring our Lord to the sick. In many cases, these ministers are old in years. Even though God may have called them later in the "work day" of life, they bear much fruit by their holy work. In turn, they receive the full day's wages due to our Lord's mercy. Likewise, those who are infirm with cancer may also toil vigorously in the Lord's vineyard even amidst their sufferings. Their efforts may be offered in union with their prayers and acts of love for others. Such souls may also receive a full day's wages from the Lord no matter what time they respond to His call in life.

Work is a blessing from God that allows us to respond to His mercy and love with gratitude and adoration. Those who suffer from cancer may not be able to maintain employment. This may be due to weakness, an inability to concentrate, or from the need for frequent medical treatments, appointments, and hospitalizations. However, they may always work in the Lord's vineyard, laboring for the Master. Such degrees of service may allow one to reach great levels of sanctity as they glorify God and help establish His kingdom here on earth.

Many of us like to see the fruits of our labors from any work we do in life. This includes our spiritual toil. We have been told that our Lord uses some individuals to sow the seeds of faith. Others are used to water the seeds. Still others are sent to help reap the harvest. As such, those who plant or later water often never see the fruit of the harvest.

Jesus told St. Faustina, **It should be of no concern to you how anyone else acts; you are to be My living reflection, through love and mercy.** Saint Faustina responded, "Lord, but they often take advantage of my goodness." Jesus then told her, **That makes no difference, My daughter. That is no concern of yours. As for you, be always merciful toward other people and especially toward sinners** (*Diary*, 1446).

Healthcare providers who care for those with cancer should use the gifts of mercy and love given by Almighty God. This call of ministry is not only for priests and religious. Every day, as patients are cured from otherwise fatal cancers, the Lord's Word is fulfilled. Some patients have tumors removed through the hands of skillful surgeons. Other cancer patients may receive effective radiation therapy to eliminate their disease. Others require chemotherapy or other treatments from their hematologist or oncologist to help eradicate their diseases.

Josh was a man who had acute leukemia. He presented with bleeding in his brain. His survival was in doubt. His wife, Pat, was horrified and remained closely at his side. Josh may have died rapidly had he not received numerous blood and platelet transfusions as well as therapy for his cancer. After such treatment, he achieved a remission from his disease. With further therapy and supportive care, Josh continued to recover.

As of this writing, many years later, he is alive and well with his disease cured. He eventually returned to work and to his normal daily routine. Life, though, was not the same for Josh after this experience. His job and family were the same as before his illness, but he had a new outlook on life. As he performed daily tasks, they had new meaning. He could use each of them as an opportunity to serve God and others. Josh's new life reflected the profound gratitude he had for those who helped care for him through the Lord's grace and mercy.

When healthcare professionals work together, wonderful things can happen. As in other walks of life, disputes, animosity, power struggles, and jealousy must be shunned, for such conduct is destructive. These temptations can be overcome by prayer, fasting, humility, and allowing the Holy Spirit to work in our lives. God's mercy transcends human weakness and allows unity through love and mutual respect.

Saint Faustina recorded words from Our Blessed Mother, who told her, *Oh, how pleasing to God is the soul that follows faithfully the inspirations of His grace! I gave the Savior to the world; as for you, you have to speak to the world about His great mercy and prepare the world for the Second Coming of Him who will come, not as a merciful Savior, but as a just Judge. Oh, how terrible is that day! Determined is the day of justice, the day of divine wrath. The angels tremble before it. Speak to souls about this great mercy while it is still the time for [granting] mercy. If you keep silent now, you will be answering for a great number of souls on that terrible day. Fear nothing. Be faithful to the end. I sympathize with you* (*Diary*, 635).

As I make hospital rounds, I go room to room to see different patients and to assess their clinical conditions. Each day as I enter patients' rooms and evaluate them, I may have either good or bad news to tell them. In some cases, patients and their families may hear their disease is not responding to treatment. I tell others that things are going well, they are recovering, or their disease is responding nicely to treatment. However, each day, patients may always receive the Good News from our Lord Jesus Christ. The message of Divine Mercy and hope should encourage us all. No matter what difficulties and struggles occur in this world or in any patient's life, these are overcome if one completely trusts in the Lord with deep faith.

Jesus also tells us you can tell a tree by its fruit. A good tree produces good fruit, while a bad tree produces rotten fruit. Similarly, a good person produces goodness from the stores of his or her heart, while an evil person produces evil (see Mt 12:35). Those who care for the sick with love bear good fruit. Our lives of service must, therefore, be rich in mercy and love.

Often fundraising events are held by cancer centers to help support patients with cancer as well as research to work for cures. A number of philanthropic organizations raise large amounts of money each year to help attain these goals. Numerous benefactors donate much of their time, talent, and financial support to make these dreams a reality.

In the Church, many people from various walks of life also contribute for the good of the kingdom and building up of the Body of Christ. Cancer patients are integral members of the Church, and their great sacrifices and suffering have beneficial effects for others. Little acts of love and kindness are routinely performed by such souls.

Two patients I cared for were Jim and Fred. They had been hospitalized in the same room as they received treatment. Although they were of much different ages and backgrounds, Jim and Fred became comrades. One day, Jim went off the floor and returned with a can of soda pop that his older roommate, Fred, had greatly desired. Such small acts of kindness performed with great love have always been building blocks within the Church as taught by many of the saints, including St. Therese of the Child Jesus, the Little Flower, and St. Josemaría Escrivá.

Luke was a cancer survivor who had been cured after much treatment and time in the hospital. As he regained his strength, he began to run. With time and practice, Luke was able to run for miles. He decided to participate in a marathon to help raise money for the Leukemia/Lymphoma Society. Like many others, Luke put this holy work ahead of his own limitations, and he trained intensely with great passion. He also traveled, and others witnessed Luke's great passion for life. He had maintained a positive attitude when dealing with others, and this also inspired them to pursue great things for God and others.

When our work may seem mundane or to count for little, we should recall that work is a blessing. When consecrated to the Lord God, it can be a pleasing sacrifice of great spiritual merit, regardless of the value it holds in the eyes of the world.

Although many healthcare providers commit their lives to the service of those with cancer, numerous patients experience difficulties obtaining the necessary medical insurance approval to get adequate coverage. Some patients have been denied medical coverage for participation in clinical trials, while others may have been unable to receive an effective therapy for their disease due to the cost of such treatment.

Thomas was a man with an advanced blood cancer who needed a bone marrow transplant, since this was the only known potential cure for his disease. However, his medical insurance coverage did not approve him for this therapy. In these situations, there is often already great anxiety for patients like Thomas who face their life-threatening diseases. To then find out that one has no way to pay for the treatment is another problem.

In the spiritual life, one does not need to wonder whether he or she will be "covered" spiritually. The Lord's mercy and love are infinite and available for all. The only prerequisite is that we come to this fount of grace with humble, contrite hearts completely trusting in God.

Sometimes caring for cancer patients does not require active treatment, yet their oncologists need to provide further health services. For instance, some patients with chronic leukemia or indolent lymphoma may be followed for years without treatment if they remain without significant symptoms or ill effects from their disease. In addition, other patients in remission after therapy for their cancers may only need regular monitoring without further treatment. Such patients often have follow-up appointments with their oncologists for physical exams, blood work, and occasionally other screening tests such as X-rays or CT scans as well. These check-ups are forms of routine maintenance intended to detect evidence of recurrent or progressive disease early on to intervene as soon as possible.

Souls in a state of grace must similarly have routine spiritual "maintenance" or "screening services" to prevent them from falling into sin. This is necessary in order for them to function properly in their service of the Lord. Regular participation in Holy Mass and reception of the Sacraments, including Reconciliation, are necessary to maintain spiritual health. Regular prayer — including silent contemplation, spiritual reading, the recitation of the Holy Rosary, the

Chaplet of The Divine Mercy, and a daily examination of conscience — are also important. These are effective means for one to excel spiritually and attain deeper states of grace and union with God.

In turn, we are all called to greater service as we hear Jesus tell us: "Without cost you have received; without cost you are to give" (Mt 10:8).

CHAPTER THREE
Thankfulness

From the Scriptures, we hear of those who were grateful to Almighty God for showing them His mercy during their lives. We recall how the Lord in His great Mercy blessed Joseph after he had been sold into slavery in Egypt. The pharaoh later gave him great wealth and placed him in charge of all Egypt as an expression of his gratitude (see Gen 37 and 41). Later, we hear of how grateful the Israelites were after they had crossed through the parted Red Sea as the Lord God delivered them from the Egyptians (see Ex 15). Others such as Naaman the Syrian wished to give the Prophet Elisha great monetary gifts after he was healed of his leprosy (see 2 Kgs 5). In the Gospels, we hear that after Zacchaeus the tax collector experienced the Lord's mercy, he went and offered large sums of repayment in reparation for his sins (see Lk 19:8). The Holy Spirit prompts such acts of gratitude after one experiences the great mercy of God.

It is astounding for me to see the profound gratitude many cancer patients show despite their challenging circumstances. They often notice the smallest things performed for them, whether it is bringing them a beverage, providing them with reading material, getting them an extra blanket, or taking time to talk with them.

On one occasion, 10 lepers came to Jesus and asked Him to have pity on them and heal them. After curing them, however, only one returned to thank Jesus (see Lk 17:11-19). Frequently, cancer patients resemble the sole leper who returns to thank our Lord. Such souls have a sincere appreciation for a second chance at life. When they give their renewed lives to the Lord, He, in turn, can grant them His peace.

Mary was one of my patients with a blood cancer. She frequently told me she was blessed. Despite the hardships she endured, she constantly thanked the healthcare team but, more importantly, Almighty God. She realized that though she suffered, this was nothing compared to what some other patients had to endure from their diseases. Mary also was aware that her difficulties were just a small reflection of what our Lord Jesus suffered for her and all people.

I find it remarkable to see that many cancer patients with a deep faith seem to require little support from others, since they have entrusted their lives to the Lord. Others may think such patients are pitiable, but in fact these patients commonly realize how much they are loved by God and, in turn, are profoundly grateful.

Although being thankful for material things is appropriate, far more important is gratitude for spiritual gifts. In particular, the gift of faith must never be taken for granted. It must be greatly treasured, nurtured, and protected throughout one's life. Patients like Mary recognize the infinite value of such faith. They also may share the joy the Apostles had when Jesus said, "But blessed are your eyes, because they see, and your ears, because they hear. Amen, I say to you many prophets and righteous people longed to see what you see but did not see it, and to hear what you hear but did not hear it" (Mt 13:16-17).

Elizabeth was a woman who suffered with horrible mouth sores that were bleeding after she had received her chemotherapy. She was unable to eat for weeks, and she required significant amounts of pain medications. Despite her suffering, Elizabeth remained continually thankful for her medical care, and she maintained a pleasant personality throughout her trying times. Moreover, she reflected a deep sense of peace through her life to others. Elizabeth's witness of Christian virtue also permeated many others' lives in order to strengthen and inspire them to great holiness as well.

Phyllis was another of my patients. She had received a bone marrow transplant for a blood condition known as a chronic myeloproliferative disorder (see Glossary). Although she had been a strong woman, after her transplant, many serious complications occurred that lead to a gradual decline in physical strength.

She developed a bowel infection that required urgent surgery, and from which she was left with a colostomy. For many months, she had as much as three to four liters of diarrhea daily. Phyllis then developed profound weakness with malnutrition that required intravenous feeding. Later, she was found to have a painful compression fracture in her lower spine. Then Phyllis developed a serious pneumonia that required resection of a portion of her lung. One problem after another continued to arise, and each one weakened Phyllis physically more and more.

In this situation, many people would complain and despair. Yet Phyllis's character and resolve were of a higher nature. Despite the many trials, her life was a continual song of gratefulness. She constantly thanked each person she encountered, even for the slightest acts of kindness. My colleagues and I were often surprised at her deep appreciation after we performed the simplest things. Such thankfulness helps others to realize how precious their acts of mercy are in the world.

Our Lord has taught us that we are never alone, for He is with us always. In particular, Jesus has sent us His Holy Spirit, who abides in us if we remain in a state of grace. When we are open to God's grace and sincerely ask Him for what we need, He will give us the greatest gift, His very self in the Holy Spirit (see Lk 11:13). He is our defender. He showers us with His infinite Mercy.

Jesus told St. Faustina, **My daughter, tell souls that I am giving them My Mercy as a defense. I Myself am fighting for them and am bearing the just anger of My Father** (*Diary*, 1516). Souls should thus be ever grateful for this wonderful gift of Divine Mercy and should continually offer songs of thanksgiving as part of their prayer.

Shirley was an older woman who had been hospitalized for weeks due to her cancer. She also at times suffered considerably. However, when I visited her one day, she expressed deep thanks.

Though I do not recall having had anything special to say that day, Shirley said my visit lifted her spirits and brought her great joy. As I reflected on that day, I remembered that it had been busy for me as I moved rapidly from one task to another. Although I had been somewhat exhausted, after my encounter with Shirley that afternoon, it was I who found my own spirit lifted and full of delight. Her few simple words spoken to me with great love left me, in turn, grateful to both her and our Lord for touching my life in the midst of its hectic pace.

Often in medicine, as in many other types of work, people do not take time to thank others. In many cases, though people may be appreciative, they are not demonstrative about this to others because they are caught up in the hustle of things. Unfortunately, many fail to slow down and reflect on how God is working in their lives.

Saint Isidore is a wonderful example of someone who took time for the Lord. Though he was responsible for plowing the land for his master, he took time to thank the Lord and express his love by attending daily Mass. When others complained he was not working the full time but instead going to Mass, his master decided to observe if this was the case. However, he found that when St. Isidore had been absent from the fields while at Mass, angels had been performing his work. Thus, when people take the necessary time to thank God for His goodness and Divine Mercy, He always provides above and beyond what they ever could have accomplished by themselves.

Some cancer patients have a deep awareness of their many blessings despite their illnesses. They show a deep appreciation to the Lord for the many things that they have received, such as being able to leave the hospital or perhaps an intensive care unit. Others who had been immobile may be grateful for later being able to walk again. Some rejoice with gratitude when they can eat or when they can breathe without an oxygen tank. These simple things we take for granted each day are wonderful gifts that our Lord gives to many of us. With daily reflection and an examination of conscience, one is able to better appreciate that these important things in life should not be taken for granted.

Frank was a lively man of high social standing. However, he developed a cancer that profoundly compromised his immune system. Frank later contracted an infection and eventually succumbed to his disease. During his hospitalization, many healthcare providers attended to him and his family.

After Frank's death, his wife and son were grateful for the care he had received. His family then carried out what they believed Frank's wishes would have been. This included a large donation of money for cancer research at our hospital. Although they may not have received any personal benefit from this gesture of gratitude, Frank's wife and son had others in mind. They knew that without resources being provided to help through research, other patients with Frank's cancer would also die.

Many others, including cancer survivors, have shared this same passion for life. In particular, those cured of their diseases tend to be extremely thankful. They often look for ways to assist others with cancer. This may be through financial assistance, actions to physically support the sick, or simply words of encouragement and concern. Hence, gratitude prompts such individuals to act. They are inspired to show others compassion and to live like Jesus Christ.

Tom was an older patient I came to know well over time. He had been successfully treated for an aggressive lymphoma, but he continued to follow up with me for years afterward. He joked with me routinely at each of these visits. Tom was naturally grateful to be cured from his cancer. He let me know he did not have much monetary wealth. However, Tom told me that if he came across any he would make a large donation to our cancer center for medical care and research.

Cancer patients commonly display tremendous gratitude to others for the love they have been shown, but this does not require donations of money. Far more important is that patients like Tom develop loving hearts patterned after those of the saints.

CHAPTER FOUR

Patience, Perseverance, and Cultivating Silence

Those with cancer have the opportunity to purify their hearts and grow in great virtue. In particular, many such souls have been blessed with tremendous patience as they learn to persevere even in the most trying circumstances. In many cases, these gifts have been granted and perfected over a period of time. Just as people pray for the grace to be patient and persevere, so the Lord often provides them with opportunities to attain these virtues. If everything went smoothly all the time, how could we expect to become more patient? If there were not challenges, how could we grow in perseverance? The Lord knows what each of us needs to advance in holiness. As our loving Father, He grants us the grace necessary to develop our spiritual lives in the manner that He best sees fit. We need only to trust in Him.

The Lord also provides us with the gift of faith that allows us to receive everlasting life. Each of us must greatly treasure this awesome gift throughout our lives. Furthermore, we need to make it a living faith, which is actively practiced, so we can preserve it and foster its growth.

Jesus helps us understand the importance of waiting patiently and being well prepared for His return. He said, "Gird your loins and light your lamps and be like servants who await their master's return from a wedding, ready to open immediately when he comes and knocks. Blessed are those servants whom the master finds vigilant on his arrival. Amen, I say to you, he will gird himself, have them recline at table, and proceed to wait on them. And should he come in the second or third watch and find them prepared in this way, blessed are those servants" (Lk 12:35-38).

As we contemplate God's deep love for humankind throughout history, it is clear how patient He has been. He is a loving Father who desires perfect unity among His children, yet our sinfulness disturbs this natural order. Warfare, hate, envy, malice, lust, and other vices tarnish the beauty of God's creation. However, the Lord still remains faithful despite our lack of gratitude and love for Him. God constantly calls each of us back, and He awaits our return with the greatest possible patience. He repeatedly invites each of us to His heavenly banquet. Moreover, Jesus lived His life in this world to illustrate how to persevere in holiness. Christ shows us how we are to conquer the world.

The many holy men and women throughout history who have followed Jesus' example of love were able to grow in patience and persevere in their struggles. Those with cancer may obtain peace as they reflect on the remarkable patience of Job in the Old Testament, who remained faithful to Almighty God despite many trials. He blessed the Lord's most Holy Name as he endured numerous major calamities that included the death of his children, illness, and the loss of most of his personal possessions. Throughout the New Testament, we then hear of the marvelous witnesses of the Apostles and the early Church as they persevered in holiness despite immense opposition. Today, Jesus also helps souls achieve these virtues, including those with cancer.

By reflecting on the example of holy men and women such as St. Faustina, Blessed John Paul II, and Blessed Mother Teresa of Calcutta, those with cancer may be encouraged and strengthened to likewise live mercifully to a heroic degree. Saint Faustina was entrusted with the great work of spreading the message of Divine Mercy to the world. The Lord also asked her to form a new congregation dedicated to this work. However, shortly thereafter, she became sick from tuberculosis. She endured high fevers, violent coughing, and intense abdominal pain, thinking her death was imminent.

She could not understand how it was possible to carry out the Lord's wishes because of her poor health. Beyond this, she was constantly met with rejection and suspicion from others, which drained her strength even more. Despite these obstacles, she patiently endured her sufferings. Her great trust in the Lord enabled her to persevere in completing what the Lord commanded.

Deb was a young woman with aplastic anemia (see Glossary). This is a condition characterized by an empty bone marrow that is unable to produce blood cells. If they are left untreated or do not respond to treatment, patients with this condition will ultimately die from bleeding or infection. Deb, a single mother, underwent a bone marrow transplant, but unfortunately due to a complication (graft versus host disease, see Glossary), she suffered greatly and eventually died.

Graft versus host disease occurs after such transplants when some of the new blood cells derived from the donor (the graft) attack parts of the patient's body (the host). This complication may be prevented or successfully treated with certain medications that suppress the immune system. However, patients who do not respond to such follow-up treatment can experience significant suffering and death.

Deb spent the last several months of her life in the hospital, where she received many blood and platelet transfusions. She also received other continuous, supportive care measures to maintain her life. Unlike many other young people who may act with impulsiveness, Deb displayed remarkable patience amid her many trials. Whether she was stuck for blood draws, awakened for medical tests, examined by multiple healthcare professionals during the day, or waiting to be transported throughout the hospital, she maintained a deep sense of calm.

Deb learned to take one day at a time and not worry about the future. In doing so, she reminded me of Jesus' words, "Do not worry about tomorrow; tomorrow will take care of itself. Sufficient for a day is its own evil" (Mt 6:34). Undoubtedly, Deb wondered how her daughter would be cared for in her absence. Fortunately, her sister was supportive and took on much of this responsibility. Deb could not eat and grew weaker over time. Despite receiving intravenous nutrition, she still had to struggle to survive. Nonetheless, she patiently endured her cross each day. Although medications couldn't control her disease, Deb's deep faith and love for God provided her the serenity of spirit that helped her to triumph in the end.

Additional virtues may be perfected in the lives of other patients with cancer. Some who tend to be abrupt learn how to practice patience and kindness. Offering up inconveniences and suffering each day has enabled many to attain great sanctity. These souls wonderfully portray the true meaning of love as described by St. Paul. "Love is patient, love is kind. It is not jealous, [love] is not pompous, it is not inflated, it is not rude, it does not seek its own interests, it is not quick-tempered, it does not brood over injury, it does not rejoice over wrongdoing but rejoices with the truth. It bears all things, believes all things, hopes all things, endures all things" (1 Cor 13:4-7).

We also learn from those with religious vocations the beauty of the vow of chastity. This is a deep expression of love for God that requires one to persevere in purity.

Though the temptations she faced were difficult at times, St. Faustina wrote, "To conquer interior temptations with the thought of the presence of God, and moreover to fight without fear. And for exterior temptations, to avoid occasions. There are seven principal means: to guard the senses, to avoid occasions, to avoid idleness, to remove temptations promptly, to remove oneself from all (especially particular) friendships, the spirit of mortification, and to reveal all of these temptations to one's confessor. Besides this, there are also five means of preserving this virtue: humility, the spirit of prayer, modesty of the eyes, fidelity to the rule, a sincere devotion to the Blessed Virgin Mary" (*Diary*, 93).

These means are not only extremely useful for religious but also for the laity, including those who are married. Many cancer patients and their spouses are faced with an inability to have sexual relations. For some, this occurs due to sterilization as a side effect of chemotherapy, while for others this results from physical weakness and frailty from their disease or treatment. Others may have profound psychological effects from their illness that lead to a loss of interest in sex. This may be particularly challenging for their healthy spouses, since they must practice chastity.

Bill and Stacey, a married couple, experienced this first-hand. Although they were both young and may have wanted more children, Stacey came down with a fatal cancer. The disease progressed, and she became weaker. Though she tried to maintain her pleasant personality with others, her illness affected her relationship with Bill. In her condition, marital intimacy was no longer possible. This challenged Bill to embrace chastity for the love of his wife. Despite the great sacrifice, he had the opportunity to practice this virtue and grow in holiness.

Maintaining cheerfulness is often difficult during an illness. Betty was a woman who developed many complications after her cancer therapy, but she maintained a pleasant attitude. She had a good sense of humor despite the hardships she experienced. Even when she had to miss her son's wedding because of a hospitalization, she did not complain. Betty told me her mind often ran constantly, thinking about the uncertainties in her life. However, with perseverance and prayer, she was able to overcome one obstacle after another. Her cheerful manner became a source of strength to others. Betty's great patience amidst the many trials resulted from her faith in God. Such souls of great virtue inspire me during my life as well. Their examples of perseverance teach me to be patient when I have to wait for things.

Those with cancer may often use their time of illness to develop a deep prayer life. Through this holy practice, they may find the strength and courage to cope with any difficulty. Some people find that their lives before cancer were filled with tremendous activity, with little or no time for reflection or conversation with God. Yet with the development of cancer, many face death. In this setting, they may come to realize the gifts they have received from God and how much they treasure them. Many find this to be a time when they can listen closely to the everlasting Word of God. The Catholic Church teaches that this Word is Jesus Christ, to whom all the Scriptures point.

By reflecting on the Old and New Testaments, we find the Word of God alive throughout history. From these sacred verses, we can come to know the Lord's holy will. Bill was one of many cancer patients who recognized that the Holy Bible was his source of consolation and truth in the face of suffering. He read the Holy Scriptures intently and reflected on the various prophets, disciples, saints, Our Blessed Mother, and our Lord Jesus. From Scripture, Bill found healing, strength, and peace.

Bill had to be hospitalized. There were days when he felt weak and others when he had fevers. Beyond his physical suffering, he also missed being home with his family. He fought periodic depression. As I spoke with Bill, he shared the importance of prayer in his life. It seemed that everything he did began with prayer. He thought of prayer as a dialogue with God.

As in any relationship where two people love each other, both must be attentive to the other person. God is omnipotent, being our Creator, Redeemer, and Sanctifier. Since He loves us beyond comprehension, we must all the more continually focus every moment of our lives on loving Him in return. Therefore, our time with God should not be limited to only periods of formal prayer. Instead, we should strive to have a constant awareness of His divine presence with us throughout every moment of our lives.

Like many others with cancer, Bill had lived an active life, being assertive amidst the noise of this world. However, he came to appreciate his time with cancer as a period of quiet. From Bill's example, I was inspired to search for such silence each day. I recalled from the Gospels how Jesus would take time away from others to pray. Sometimes this necessitated Him going up a mountain or staying up all night while His disciples were asleep.

From Christ's example, we should restructure our lives. Although many have families and jobs that take much of our time, it is important to stop and reflect throughout the day, even if this is only for brief moments at a time. Those who ask the Lord will receive the quiet time that they need each day.

Saint Faustina wrote of the importance of these opportunities: "... in order to hear the voice of God, one has to have silence in one's soul and to keep silence ... that is to say, recollection in God. One can speak a great deal without breaking silence and, on the contrary, one can speak little and be constantly breaking silence. Oh, what irreparable damage is done by the breach of silence! We cause a lot of harm to our neighbor, but even more to our own selves. ... A soul that has never tasted the sweetness of inner silence is a restless spirit which disturbs the silence of others. I have seen many souls in the depths of hell for not having kept their silence. ... My God, what an agony it is to think that not only might they have been in heaven, but they might even have become saints! O Jesus, have mercy!" (*Diary*, 118).

Blessed Mother Teresa of Calcutta also taught the importance of silence. She observed that silence leads to prayer. This results in faith, which brings a person to love. The fruit of this love is service, which ushers in peace (see Mother Teresa, *Loving Jesus*, pp. 79-80).

By taking time to reflect on the people he encountered and on the events that transpired throughout each day, Bill began to see the Lord at work in his life and in the world. It has been said that after we die, we will b e amazed to see how close God was with us throughout our mortal lives. Cancer patients like Bill may come to realize this more fully as they see the face of God in their spouses, children, parents, other relatives, and friends. By examining their consciences each evening, such souls may learn great truths from the Lord by recalling their interactions with others. This knowledge, in turn, allows them to help build the kingdom of God on earth.

When I was in my early medical training, one of my teachers stated that when things do not look right or make sense from test results, go back to the patient. At their bedside, with further examination and assessment, you will usually find the answer. In this busy world we live in, as we chase from one thing to another, we often will not find the answer to the important things in life. These essential things are none other than the experience of God's mercy and our salvation from Jesus our Lord and Savior. By taking time to slow down and listen, as in the case of spending time with a patient, the Lord often reveals Himself to us. In silence, one may hear the soft whisper with which God speaks.

This was apparent in the days of the Prophet Elijah when the Lord asked him to stand on the mountain before Him. "A strong and heavy wind was rending the mountains and crushing rocks before the Lord, but the Lord was not in the wind. After the wind there was an earthquake, but the Lord was not in the earthquake. After the earthquake there was fire, but the Lord was not in the fire. After the fire there was a tiny whispering sound. When he heard this, Elijah hid his face in his cloak and went and stood at the entrance of the cave" (1 Kgs 19:11-13).

In addition to those with cancer, their families must also learn patience. Brian was a gentleman who did well after having intense chemotherapy for his blood cancer. After eliminating his disease, he was still required to be on steroids for many months. Although steroids are an effective treatment to suppress inflammation, they have considerable side effects. This is particularly true for those patients who continue to receive these drugs on a long-term basis. As Brian remained on this medication, his face and neck became swollen. He also had recurrent infections that required treatment. Beyond this, the steroid medication had major effects on Brian's mood.

Like many others, he became irritable while on this treatment. Brian would have outbursts of anger when his children did minor things that annoyed him. He also found that while taking steroids, he could not sleep well, and this undoubtedly contributed to his altered mood.

Brian's wife, Melissa, was a wonderful support for him, particularly as he received cancer treatment. However, she had much to bear when faced with his outbursts and lack of patience. The time of Brian's illness was an opportunity for Melissa as well, for she not only had to continue caring for their children, but she also had to be Brian's primary caregiver at home. Melissa encouraged him each day to get up and walk. She also assisted him with his medications and brought him back for outpatient visits. Other times, Melissa would just sit and listen to him when he was frustrated and needed to talk. This daily giving of self allowed Melissa to grow in holiness.

Small things performed with love enable people to accomplish great things as they grow in patience and perseverance.

CHAPTER FIVE

Diligence

For those with cancer, successful outcomes occur more frequently when they remain steadfast as they undergo treatment. I often tell patients that they are the center of the medical team, and their hearts must be completely into whatever plan of treatment we decide to pursue. Such dedication is necessary if a patient is to have any hope of eradicating his or her disease. Although physicians may formulate treatment plans, the patient has to come back and forth to the medical facility for check-ups and treatments. They also must follow their physicians' instructions closely to deal with side effects and help prevent other problems that can develop after receiving cancer therapies.

John had intestinal bleeding from his cancer. Fortunately, after many blood and platelet transfusions were administered, the bleeding stopped. He then received several cycles of intense chemotherapy while he remained hospitalized. John adapted well to his illness, and he realized he must fight hard every day.

Early during his treatment, he had a large catheter placed in his chest. This gave him the intravenous access necessary to receive chemotherapy, further blood products, and other medications. Each day, either John or a nurse would meticulously clean around the catheter in his chest to help prevent it from getting infected. This type of catheter has an indwelling portion that extends just above the first chamber of the heart. If such a catheter were to get infected, it could also affect the heart valves. Furthermore, patients can develop blood clots around their catheters, which then sometimes have to be removed. Therefore, patients and nurses must work diligently to keep these catheters functioning well.

Just as John needed to care for his catheter to prevent ill effects on his heart, souls must also be diligent to prevent evil from affecting their hearts. Jesus warned us to "... stay awake! For you do not know on which day your Lord will come. Be sure of this: if the master of the house had known the hour of night when the thief was coming, he would have stayed awake and not let his house be broken into. So too, you also must be prepared, for at an hour you do not expect, the Son of Man will come" (Mt 24:42-44).

Like most cancer patients, John was concerned about maintaining his quality of life. Although some with cancer will undergo any treatment or put up with any side effect in an effort to eradicate their disease, others will not do so. As patients live with cancer day by day, they often learn to tolerate many things. Yet as their diseases advance, many find their quality of life deteriorates.

Therefore, those who choose to receive cancer therapies hope to at least alleviate symptoms related to their illnesses. For some, this is pain, while for others it may be shortness of breath, loss of appetite, weight loss, or fatigue. Many other symptoms can occur in patients depending on what type of cancer they have and how rapidly their disease advances. John developed fevers as his disease progressed. Although his cancer failed to respond to standard therapies, he was determined to try and control his cancer even if it could not be cured. John, therefore, elected to receive experimental treatment.

In oncology as in all other areas of medicine, research continues in an effort to develop new treatments for patients like John. Such investigation helps solve unanswered problems and questions and can help discover new and improved ways to treat diseases. To accomplish these goals and to fund their work, investigators submit proposals and grants for financial support from the government (for example, the National Institute of Health), companies, and foundations. Researchers often submit more than one grant proposal at a time and periodically every few years to help secure the necessary funds to continue their work. The process necessitates much discipline and perseverance to be successful.

As people give their lives to the Lord to help establish His kingdom, there must also be intense planning, constancy, and discipline. The goal is not a finite sum of money that will be spent in a short period of time. Instead, our purpose is to accomplish the work of God, which has everlasting value. Souls advance spiritually through contemplative prayer, reception of the Sacraments, Eucharistic Adoration, and spiritual reading. Further growth in holiness occurs with acts of penance and reparation. It is also important to consecrate all that one does to Almighty God in union with the celebration of Holy Mass each day. It is critical to develop a plan of life for our spiritual formation. This should be our main priority in life. In doing so, we will be set free from sin and evil, and find no challenge or cross impossible to bear.

Since many cancers have unsatisfactory treatments with no known potential for cure, for decades, hematologists and oncologists have designed clinical trials to develop new therapies. Generally, drugs are developed for clinical use through three phases of clinical trials. When a promising drug is effective against cancer cells in laboratory experiments, it may then be investigated in suitable patients.

The first stage of testing is called a phase I trial. The purpose of this trial is to determine the best dose of the drug for patients. Early in the trial, patients receive the lowest planned starting dose, and they are monitored closely for side effects. If the first group of patients on the trial tolerate the therapy well, additional patients receive a higher dose of the treatment drug. Phase I trials often continue this dose escalation until significant side effects are noted. From this experience, patients also are followed closely to determine if their cancers are responding to the treatment.

If a drug is tolerable, it can then be further investigated. This second stage of drug development is called a phase II clinical trial. Typically, phase II trials use the best-recommended dose of a drug that was determined from the phase I trial to determine how active the agent actually is against a specific type of cancer.

If the drug shows a significant number of responses, it may then be compared with the prior best standard treatment for that particular cancer in a phase III trial. In general for these trials, half of the patients receive the prior standard therapy and the other half receive the new drug. Patients are then monitored closely to assess differences between the treatments. If the new drug proves more effective, and particularly if it prolongs survival, it may then become the new standard therapy.

Our spiritual life can also go through similar phases of development. Extreme diligence is necessary to help one advance to higher stages of spirituality. In the early stages, small trials may be encountered to test one's faith. As in the case of a phase I clinical trial for cancer patients, the trial proceeds to the next higher dose level if there are no significant or intolerable side effects observed among the first group of patients. Likewise, challenges in the spiritual life may increase as the soul overcomes small struggles. This, in turn, results in further endurance and spiritual growth. During a phase I clinical trial, patients are assessed for responses against their cancer.

If responses are observed and the drug can be administered at an acceptable dose without intolerable side effects, plans are often made to design a phase II trial. During our spiritual journey in this life, individuals advance to higher levels of grace as they overcome prior obstacles by God's goodness and His Divine Mercy.

In the setting of a phase II trial for drug development, doctors want to see consistently good responses against a disease to demonstrate that the drug is effective. In the course of one's spiritual life, it is also imperative that there are consistently "good responses." These are manifested as Christian love of God and neighbor, plus works of mercy.

The soul that carries out our Lord's work during this life on earth ultimately advances to the final phase of spiritual development. Here one must choose whether or not to completely commit his or her life to the Lord for the sake of His kingdom.

In this final trial, the two things being compared are life in Christ for eternity versus eternal death. Just as a cancer therapy has to successfully advance through development prior to final testing, the soul must also advance from prior trials to be ready for the final trial in life.

At the end of a phase III trial of cancer therapy, conclusions are made as to whether the therapy was better, worse, or the same as the prior standard therapy. At the conclusion of the soul's final journey, the Lord will also be able to judge whether the person was better, worse, or the same as when they started their life. Jesus describes this in the parable of the master who left different amounts of talents with each of his three servants before he departed on a journey. The first two servants were prudent and invested the talents to return their master's money with interest. They were rewarded and received greater responsibility. However, the third servant buried his master's talents and returned this same amount back to him upon his return. The master had that servant's talents taken away, and he was expelled for not using his gifts (see Mt 25:14-30).

Another important aspect of any clinical trial is the need for patients to give informed consent prior to enrolling in a program. The risks, benefits, and alternatives of the treatment must be presented clearly to patients. They must also demonstrate a good understanding of these before the investigational therapy begins.

Likewise, in the spiritual life, a soul must freely consent to follow the teachings of Jesus and to willingly embrace the various trials it will encounter to advance in grace and holiness. Just as cancer patients cannot be forced to receive treatment, God does not force souls to lead lives of faith. Rather, individuals have a free will that they exercise to choose right or wrong.

In the case of infants and children with cancer, their parents or legal guardians consent for them to receive medical care. In some cases, this may include participation on a clinical trial. More importantly, for spiritual matters pertaining to such little ones, the elderly, or mentally infirm, it is necessary for their caregivers or responsible guardians to consent appropriately on

214 | Divine Mercy, Triumph over Cancer

their behalf. The individuals responsible for their care must be committed to bring these souls up in the Catholic faith. They must also help provide them with the spiritual nourishment necessary to advance in holiness.

All members of the Catholic Church have an obligation to not only progress in their own but also to assist in the spiritual life of others. Such commitment is integral to advancing God's kingdom.

CHAPTER SIX

Growing in Trust

Various challenges occur in the lives of those with cancer. These may include a new cancer diagnosis, progression of their disease, toxicity from therapy, strained or broken relationships, and other difficulties. However, the Lord tells us to come to Him amidst the storms and rough waters of our lives. We must completely trust in Him and His infinite mercy lest we perish. If we falter, we should know that Jesus is always waiting to help us. We must learn to be quiet and still. Those who trust in God may then experience a great calm, which comes about in the midst of these storms during life.

Faith is a critical part of many cancer patients' lives. Faith allows God to work wonders through them. Alice was a woman with breast cancer that had spread throughout her body. She received chemotherapy, but this was not as effective as she hoped. Despite her illness, she maintained a deep prayer life that she wished to share with her children, who had drifted away from the faith. Alice continued to plead with family members and friends to repent of their sins, return to the Sacraments, go to Mass, and to show mercy and love. Although Alice's words of truth were often ignored, she deeply believed in the mercy of God. She entrusted her loved ones who had fallen away to the merciful Heart of Christ.

Jesus told us the parable of the widow who kept bringing her case before the unjust judge. This judge said that he cared little for God or other men, but the widow wore him out, and he gave in to her wishes. Our Lord told us to learn from this parable. If we, in turn, petition God, who is good, how much more will He give to us? Jesus then asked, "But when the Son of Man returns will He find faith on the earth?" (see Lk 18:1-8).

As we reflect on these words, it becomes clear that we must have great trust in Him and not just continually ask for one thing after another until we get our way.

It is also important to understand that we often do not know how to pray as we should. Rather than just praying for the petitions we desire, we should ask Our Blessed Mother and the Holy Spirit to help form our prayers that they may be sincere and pleasing to Almighty God. As such, those with cancer or their loved ones who are praying for them need not worry of their own insufficiencies during prayer. They need only to approach the Lord with a contrite spirit, completely trusting in His infinite mercy and goodness. Then they will receive the grace needed to do God's holy will and to be pleasing to Him.

Saint Faustina is a wonderful example of one who trusted the Lord. From a young age, she wanted to enter the convent, but her parents did not wish her to do so. She clearly heard the Lord's persistent call for her to pursue the religious life. She had no idea at first how she was to accomplish this goal, for she had a limited education and no financial means to pursue such a vocation. As she left home and visited one convent after another, she met rejection. However, St. Faustina did not despair. Rather, she trusted that the Lord would accomplish His purpose in her life.

Eventually, she was accepted to the Sisters of Our Lady of Mercy. Throughout her time in the convent, she experienced many private revelations by the Lord. The Lord's commands were difficult at times, and she did not know how she could accomplish them.

For instance, Jesus requested that she have His sacred image painted for others to venerate. She had no skills to paint, though, and she did not know anyone who could complete this work. Still, she remained confident that Jesus' desire would be accomplished. Shortly thereafter, with the help of her spiritual director, Blessed Fr. Michael Sopocko, St. Faustina was able to meet with a painter who performed the holy work.

Likewise, when later faced with uncertainties as to how she could spread The Divine Mercy message and start a new congregation while suffering from tuberculosis, she simply trusted Christ's words. Her remarkable witness has since helped change the world by assisting countless souls to trust in Jesus.

Our Lord told St. Faustina, **My daughter, write the greater the misery of a soul, the greater its right to My mercy; urge all souls to trust in the unfathomable abyss of My mercy, because I want to save them all. On the cross, the fountain of My mercy was opened wide by the lance for all souls — no one have I excluded!** (*Diary*, 1182).

In particular, those souls who immerse themselves completely in Jesus' mercy, adoring it and glorifying it, are pleasing to the Lord for their obedience (see *Diary*, 1572). To possess a deep confidence in the Lord is a true gift. Souls who have no doubts in God's mercy do not live in fear but rather in trust.

Saint Paul tells us, "For those who are led by the Spirit of God are children of God. For you did not receive a spirit of slavery to fall back into fear, but you received a spirit of adoption, through which we cry, Abba, Father! The Spirit itself bears witness with our spirit that we are children of God, and if children, then heirs, heirs of God and joint heirs with Christ, if only we suffer with Him so that we may also be glorified with Him" (Rom 8:14-17).

I will never forget a young woman named Stacey. She and her husband just found out that she was pregnant, and they were joyful as they awaited the birth of their child. However, Stacey soon learned she had melanoma, an aggressive form of skin cancer that can spread rapidly. This disease is resistant to most treatments once it spreads out of the skin. Stacey was referred to an oncologist at the University of Chicago, who I was working with during my training. This provided me the opportunity to get to know this remarkable woman.

After her initial visit to our clinic, she had a chest X-ray performed that identified a lung nodule. This indicated that her disease had spread systemically and was, therefore, incurable. However, Stacey was only in her first trimester of pregnancy at the time. Any aggressive treatments for her disease may have resulted in either a spontaneous abortion of her child or potentially significant birth defects. Although some other patients may have sought an abortion to proceed with therapies for their cancer, Stacey did not consider this an option. Her only goal was to allow the child in her womb to have time to develop, so she could have a successful delivery. Her trust in God was remarkable, and it clearly had an effect on others.

As I watched Stacey and her husband suffer, my heart was pierced with sorrow. I prayed to God, asking why this had to happen to her. Then from a Gospel reading, I heard the Lord respond to me. Jesus was speaking to His disciples and said "... that He must go to Jerusalem and suffer greatly from the elders, the chief priests and the scribes, and be killed and on the third day be raised. Then Peter took Him aside and began to rebuke Him, 'God forbid, Lord! No such thing shall ever happen to you.' He turned and said to Peter, 'Get behind Me, Satan! You are an obstacle to Me. You are thinking not as God does, but as human beings do'" (Mt 16:21-23). I then realized Stacey's sufferings might have been the cross she was given to bear to best glorify Almighty God.

My attitude changed from one of fear for her to one of deeper compassion and love. It became clear that even if I could not help bring about a cure, I certainly could help Stacey carry her cross by trying my best to be a caring and dedicated physician as well as a brother in Christ who loved her and her family. Since that time, I have tried to remember this valuable lesson of mercy as I have cared for many others suffering from cancer.

Fear may sometimes surface as patients are diagnosed with a cancer or are faced with difficult treatment decisions and potential side effects. In addition, others may have significant concerns if their diseases recur after prior treatment. We must always hold fast to Jesus' command not to fear, for He is with us always. Such trust allows one to endure and overcome the many trials and difficulties in life.

During St. Faustina's time of suffering, she prayed to Jesus, saying, "Lord, I doubt that You will pardon my numerous sins; my misery fills me with fright."

However, Jesus then replied, **My mercy is greater than your sins and those of the entire world. Who can measure the extent of My goodness? For you I descended from heaven to earth; for you I allowed Myself to be nailed to the cross; for you I let My Sacred Heart be pierced with a lance, thus opening wide the source of mercy for you. Come, then, with trust to draw graces from this fountain. I never reject a contrite heart. Your misery has disappeared in the depths of My mercy. Do not argue with Me about your wretchedness. You will give me pleasure if you hand over to Me all your troubles and griefs. I shall heap upon you the treasures of My grace** (*Diary*, 1485).

Steve was a gentleman who had a relapse of his aggressive cancer. As such, he knew that his death would come soon. At times, Steve seemed petrified, and he continued to be extremely concerned about his future. Many people have similar concerns and anxieties in life, often over far less significant things. However, Jesus tells us, "Amen, amen, I say to you, unless a grain of wheat falls to the ground and dies, it remains just a grain of wheat; but if it dies, it produces much fruit. Whoever loves his life loses it, and whoever hates his life in this world will preserve it for eternal life" (Jn 12:24-25).

Although it was difficult for Steve to face death, many people offered him prayers, encouragement, and support, from which he experienced healing. In particular, as his wife, Rose, came to his side, she held his hands in a gesture of great love. Steve's courage seemed to increase, and he was able to go on with his life. By showing such mercy and love, we, too, can transform other souls who fear and help increase their trust in God.

Our Lord also taught St. Faustina the powerful prayer, O Blood and Water, which gushed forth from the Heart of Jesus as a fount of Mercy for us, I trust in You (*Diary*, 187). Jesus said, **When you say this prayer, with a contrite heart and with faith on behalf of some sinner, I will give him the grace of conversion** (*Diary*, 186).

We should not doubt the power of our Lord's Word.

Instead, we are to invoke His mercy not only for ourselves but others. Although many souls suffer terribly from cancer, far more suffer much worse from sin that remains in their hearts. As we trust in Jesus and invoke His grace, we may help bring about the everlasting healing the world so greatly needs.

Jesus also told St. Faustina, **Mankind will not have peace until it turns with trust to My mercy. Oh, how much I am hurt by a soul's distrust! Such a soul professes that I am Holy and Just, but does not believe that I am Mercy and does not trust in My Goodness. Even the devils glorify My Justice but do not believe in My Goodness. My Heart rejoices in this title of Mercy** (*Diary*, 300).

Fidelity to the Lord is crucial, for it is the means by which one stays in a state of grace. However, for those who stray, there is still great hope if they seek the Lord's limitless mercy. We hear Jesus tell us in the Gospel, "... ask and you will receive; seek and you will find; knock and the door will be opened to you" (Lk 11:9). Although Jesus' tremendous mercy and love are being poured out continually upon the world, we have to be open and receptive to receive such graces. If one even makes the slightest effort, the Lord's mercy and grace can accomplish unimaginable things. As a soul progresses in holiness it asks, seeks, and knocks more and more. In turn, the Lord fills such trusting souls more and more with His grace manifested by His infinite mercy and love.

One family had a young son, Casey, who was found during Holy Week 2005 to have a severely low count in his white blood cells. The findings were suspicious for a potential leukemia. Casey's parents naturally were filled with anxiety. The child was evaluated by a pediatric hematologist/oncologist, who planned to perform a bone-marrow examination the next day. Meanwhile, Casey needed to be stuck with a needle for blood draws. Like many other children, he was terrified of needles.

As Casey's parents watched him struggle from fear, they tried with the medical staff to console him. They knew well that despite the brief suffering he would experience, the intention of the medical team was only for good. With time and many words of encouragement, Casey began to trust the medical staff. He then allowed them to obtain the needed tests.

Casey's father then reflected on how Our Most Blessed Mother watched in agony while her own Son's most Sacred hands and feet were being pierced by the nails of the cross. This was performed due to the hatred and sin of humankind with no good intention for her child. Jesus, though, turned this evil into good as He offered this suffering up for our salvation.

The evening of Holy Thursday, Casey's father attended the Liturgy of the Lord's Supper. He placed his trust in God that the Lord's most holy will would be done.

At the closing of the Mass, the Most Blessed Sacrament was being carried by the priest through the church to be reposed until the Easter Vigil. As the procession came by, Casey's father bowed in reverence before the Lord. His thoughts were then focused on Jesus' heavenly Father, who knew that His Son would suffer terribly during His Passion and later die a horrible death. He prayed that he would have the courage to allow God's will to be accomplished regarding his own son, Casey.

The next day, Good Friday, the family went to see the child's physician, who ran further blood tests. They were informed that Casey's blood counts had significantly improved and that there was no evidence of leukemia. The family thanked God for His great mercy and love, while reflecting on how God the Father still allowed His own Son to die instead for the salvation of all.

As Casey's family rejoiced, his father wished to proclaim the Lord's mercy to everyone. His progress seemed slow, particularly when others did not share his enthusiasm for such mercy. If people proclaim the Word of God and are not well received or if they see no fruit from their labors, they should not lose hope. To remain steadfast in faith, it is imperative that no matter how trying our circumstances may be, we should not lose hope. Rather, we should trust all the more. Our focus should remain on praying continually for Divine Mercy and placing all things in the Lord's hands.

How many countless saints have done so without know-ing at the time the effect of their prayers and offerings? Some have prayed for a sick loved one with cancer to repent and return to the Lord's open arms, which await the person with His mercy. Although the conversion of some such people is outwardly apparent, for others only in the depths of their souls does such conversion occur before death. Regardless, God's holy will is accomplished as His lost sheep return home to His flock.

Saint Faustina wrote, "I often attend upon the dying and through entreaties obtain for them trust in God's mercy, and I implore God for an abundance of divine grace, which is always victorious. God's mercy sometimes touches the sinner at the last moment in a wondrous and mysterious way. Outwardly, it seems as if everything were lost, but it is not so. The soul illumined by a ray of God's powerful final grace, turns to God in the last moment with such a power of love that, in an instant, it receives from God forgiveness of sin and punishment, while outwardly it shows no sign either of repentance or of contrition, because souls [at that stage] no longer react to external things. Oh, how beyond comprehension is God's mercy!" (*Diary*, 1698).

Saint Faustina also noted in horror that there are still souls that reject this grace. However, she also wrote, "Although a person is at the point of death, the merciful God gives the soul that interior vivid moment, so that if the soul is willing, it has the possibility of returning to God" (*Diary*, 1698).

Some cancer patients and their families have had their relationships seriously challenged. Sally was one such individual. She underwent tremendous hardships after having a bone marrow transplant for leukemia. During this time, she was depressed and lacked confidence. Many physicians, nurses, and other healthcare providers kept trying to encourage her as she received her treatment.

Sally gradually became stronger as she responded to the therapy. Thankfully, she recovered and was cured. However, during her illness, her husband left her. Sally also had a young daughter who needed to be raised. Because of her illness, Sally had been unable to work, but fortunately her mother offered assistance during this time of great trial.

Despite this tragedy in Sally's family life, she grew immensely from these experiences. She embraced her new life without cancer and without her husband. She learned to trust. Sally was also eventually able to support her daughter through the Spirit of the Lord, who helped her leave her fears behind. Similarly, all of us must live without fear of anything. As our Lord told St. Faustina, those who trust in His mercy with complete confidence are pleasing to Him and thus receive His abundant blessings.

Jesus also told St. Faustina, **Let souls who are striving for perfection particularly adore My mercy, because the abundance of graces which I grant them flows from My mercy. I desire that these souls distinguish themselves by boundless trust in My mercy. I Myself will attend to the sanctification of such souls. I will provide them with every-thing they will need to attain sanctity. The graces of My mercy are drawn by means of one vessel only, and that is — trust. The more a soul trusts, the more it will receive. Souls that trust boundlessly are a great comfort to Me, because I pour all the treasures of My graces into them. I rejoice that they ask for much, because it is My desire to give much, very much. On the other hand, I am sad when souls ask for little, when they narrow their hearts** (*Diary*, 1578).

Like Sally each of us must trust and not be afraid to ask the Lord for too much. He waits for us to turn to Him.

PART FOUR

How Those Affected by Cancer
Can Advance the Kingdom

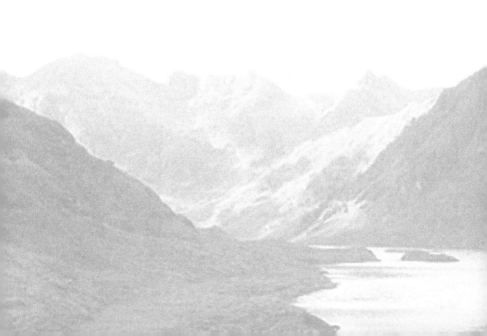

CHAPTER ONE

Showing Mercy to Others

Although we may rejoice in the Lord's mercy and infinite goodness, we must, in turn, respond with mercy toward our brothers and sisters. Jesus tells us, "Be merciful, just as your Father is merciful" (Lk 6:36).

We hear in the Gospel, "When the Son of Man comes in His glory ... He will sit upon His glorious throne, and all the nations will be assembled before Him. And He will separate them one from another, as a shepherd separates the sheep from the goats. He will place the sheep on His right and the goats on His left. Then the king will say to those on His right, 'Come, you who are blessed by My Father. Inherit the kingdom prepared for you from the foundation of the world. For I was hungry and you gave Me food, I was thirsty and you gave Me drink, a stranger and you welcomed Me, naked and you clothed Me, ill and you cared for Me, in prison and you visited Me.'" Then the righteous will ask the Lord when they did these things for Him. He will answer, "Amen, I say to you; whatever you did for one of these least brothers of mine, you did for Me." The Lord will then tell those on His left, "Depart from Me, you accursed, into the eternal fire prepared for the devil and his angels. For I was hungry and you gave Me no food, I was thirsty and you gave Me no drink, a stranger and you gave Me no welcome, naked and you gave Me no clothing, ill and in prison, and you did not care for Me." These people will then ask when they failed to do these things for the Lord. He will answer, "Amen, I say to you, what you did not do for one of these least ones, you did not do for Me." Jesus said, "... these will go off to eternal punishment, but the righteous to eternal life" (Mt 25:31-46).

Pope John Paul II wrote his encyclical *Rich in Mercy* (*Dives in Misericordia*, 1980), which discussed how Jesus' mission was centered on revealing God the Father's merciful love. Pope John Paul II wrote, "Jesus Christ taught that man not only receives and experiences the mercy of God, but that he is also called 'to practice mercy' towards others. 'Blessed are the merciful, for they shall obtain mercy' (Mt 5:7). The Church sees in these words a call to action, and she tries to practice mercy. ... Man attains to the merciful love of God, His mercy, to the extent that he himself is interiorly transformed in the spirit of that love towards his neighbor" (*Rich in Mercy*, 7).

Many people develop a fear when they hear someone has cancer. They often distance themselves from such patients due to their uncertainty of what to say to them or of what patients may ask of them. Others may feel confronted with thoughts of their own mortality when they come in contact with a person who has a potentially life-threatening illness. However, if one comes to such an individual with cancer as to Jesus Himself, he or she may experience the call to a life of great love. As Jesus portrayed to us the beautiful image of the Good Samaritan in the Gospel (see Lk 10:29-37), we, too, are called to be this sort of a caring person to our brothers and sisters who face death.

In the cancer field, many oncologists and other healthcare providers spend their lives trying to be such Good Samaritans as they strive to eradicate this disease and improve quality of life for patients. It is unsettling not to have treatment options for any patient with cancer. Evolution of new treatments has, therefore, been important to provide such patients therapeutic options, particularly when the prior available therapies have been ineffective or can have significant side effects.

A remarkable approach to treating various blood cancers is blood or bone marrow transplantation. This procedure has been significantly refined over the years from when it first became routinely performed in the 1970s. At that time, only younger patients who had a suitable donor in their family were considered for a transplant. Unfortunately, the vast majority of patients with diseases who could potentially have been cured with this procedure were either too old, medically too unfit, or without a suitable donor. Over the years, much research has been performed to make blood and bone marrow transplantation safer and more readily available.

The constant search for ways to save lives from cancer is well illustrated by describing the history of blood and bone marrow transplantation. Prior to the availability of this procedure, blood transfusions were known to help some patients with blood cancers, but their benefit was usually short-lived. As such, these individuals often required more and more blood products over time to sustain their lives. Eventually, though, these transfusions became less effective, and patients died from their diseases.

Blood is produced within the bone marrow, which resides within the hollow portion of many bones. By obtaining some marrow from healthy donors, one may be able to restore the production of good blood cells in those with various blood diseases and cure them of their illnesses. Some patients may benefit from transplant procedures using their own bone marrow (autologous transplants), while others require healthy marrow from a donor (allogeneic transplants).

Initially, transplants were performed using only bone marrow extracted with needles from the pelvic bones of donors. Later, with the evolution of technology, these early blood cells from the bone marrow cavity could be collected from the peripheral blood. Donors receive a medicine to mobilize these cells from their bone marrow, which are then collected through a catheter placed in one of their central veins. It often allows large numbers of the early blood cells from the bone marrow to be procured.

This approach results in faster recovery of patients' blood counts after the transplant procedure compared to that observed with bone marrow. However, transplants that use these cells from the peripheral blood also result in a higher incidence of a later complication called chronic graft versus host disease (see Glossary) discussed earlier. This condition causes some patients considerable discomfort and may significantly affect their quality of life. Furthermore, a number of patients who develop graft versus host disease may die from this condition. Medicines that suppress the immune system are used to treat this disease. They also are administered in advance to try and prevent its occurrence.

Historically, blood and marrow transplants could only be performed for patients who had a family member with a compatible bone marrow type. This was a significant problem for many years, since the majority of patients did not have a matched-related donor. However, by 1987, the National Marrow Donor Program was formed, and volunteer donors who were unrelated became available.

These Good Samaritans have their bone marrow types entered into a public registry. Patients who require a transplant to cure their blood diseases but who are without matched-related donors can potentially find suitable matched-unrelated donors through this registry. Previously, the outcomes after a transplant with an unrelated donor were inferior to those with a matched-related donor. With the advance of DNA testing, bone-marrow typing methods considerably improved over time, allowing for much better identification of well-matched unrelated donors. This, in turn, improved patient outcomes after transplantation with results more comparable to that observed after a blood or marrow transplant from a matched-related donor.

Despite the millions of potential unrelated donors who are available to donate blood or bone marrow for transplantation, many cancer patients who could benefit from this treatment still cannot find a suitable donor. This is due to their rare bone marrow types. Over time, though, it became clear that these transplants could be successfully performed with umbilical cord blood as an alternative donor source. After a mother delivers her child and the umbilical cord is cut, the placenta, or afterbirth, is usually discarded. Before doing so, the blood in the umbilical cord can be collected and frozen. Later, this can be thawed out and infused into patients for their transplants.

Transplants with cord blood may be successfully performed, even though they may not be well matched with patients. Limitations for this procedure include a longer time for the blood counts to recover after the transplant procedure and a greater risk of infections compared to peripheral blood or bone marrow transplantation.

Another advance in this transplant field was the development of reduced-intensity transplants. These could be performed with far less chemotherapy or radiation therapy than that administered with traditional blood or bone marrow transplants. This approach has allowed patients who are otherwise too old or medically infirm for a traditional transplant with high-dose chemotherapy to still receive potentially curative therapy for their blood diseases.

This short review of the evolution of blood and bone marrow transplantation illustrates how many researchers and healthcare providers have devoted their careers to help others in profound need. Such innovations have taken much collaboration, effort, and guidance by the Holy Spirit to save lives. Each small step that helped advance the ways these transplants were performed, as well as each demonstration of compassion for cancer patients, was an opportunity for many caregivers to show mercy.

In oncology, when patients have diseases that are not curable, the treatment goals focus particularly on optimizing quality of life. As such, palliative care is performed, often with the administration of pain medications and other measures to obtain comfort. Although this approach is appropriate for some patients, for others, it may not be. When it comes to spiritual assistance, all patients deserve to receive bountiful support from their loved ones as well as from others and the Church.

Often on oncology wards, there are many saintly people that enter patients' lives each day. These include supportive family and friends who take time out of their busy lives to be at the side of their loved ones. As some patients approach the end of their earthly lives, these loving individuals help them carry their crosses, as Simon of Cyrene helped Jesus. Other individuals such as nurses, physicians, social workers, and volunteers may imitate St. Veronica. With great love, she was moved at the sight of our Lord's agony to boldly confront evil

232 | Divine Mercy, Triumph over Cancer

and show Him compassion by wiping His face as He went to His death. Others such as priests, nuns, other religious, and Eucharistic ministers are like Our Blessed Mother, St. John, St. Mary Magdalene, and the other faithful women who remained at the foot of Jesus' cross as He was dying.

Pat was a man with an aggressive blood cancer. He faced death as he received treatment. During his time of trial, some holy sisters prayed for him and offered support to his family. With time, Pat's condition improved, and he achieved a remission from his disease. He was able to return home to be with his wife and son once again. He then enjoyed the simple things in life such as sharing a meal with others and taking walks with his family through his neighborhood. With his life restored, Pat developed a new appreciation for prayer. He had the opportunity to reflect on what is important in this world. Prior to his illness, Pat had been a successful professor of engineering at a university. He worked long hours, which limited his time with family.

While battling cancer, he witnessed great love from not only his family but from many others, including his caregivers and the holy sisters. Like many others who experience such traumatic circumstances and survive, Pat knew his life had to change. He gradually made great spiritual progress. Pat seemed to recognize that this was by no power of his own. Rather, it occurred due to the great mercy he experienced from the Lord. He could appreciate how intimately God worked through others around him. Pat was grateful for the holy sisters who prayed for him and who had been the reflection of God's mercy. Their wonderful example of intercessory prayer should inspire us all to likewise pray for the sick to invoke the Lord's mercy and healing power.

Although we may wish to emulate such individuals who care for and support the sick and the dying, cancer patients themselves are often Good Samaritans for others. As they experience illness, they may teach others who are spiritually dying to stop focusing on self and to redirect their lives to God. It is this concern for others that has transformed many with cancer to become true witnesses of Christ's mercy. Their lives preach the Gospel boldly as the Holy Spirit uses these meek and lowly souls to shame the proud and strong, who rely on their own resources rather than on God.

Some who are ill still demonstrate remarkable kindness to others. Despite their weaknesses, these individuals maintain a true sense of compassion. This enables them to live out our Lord's command to, "Do to others as you would have them do to you" (Lk 6:31). Through the virtue of temperance, cancer patients have been able to live well by using things in moderation. They avoid gluttony and wasting time to maintain a proper balance in life. For instance, some patients who have been obese find their cancers to be a means by which to limit their intake of food and thus improve their overall health.

Others with cancer have learned to offer up various mortifications which, when joined to the sufferings of Christ, are of tremendous redemptive benefit. Still other patients develop a great tolerance for those with different backgrounds. This allows them to welcome those who are strangers as Jesus commands us to do (see Mt 25:35).

Some patients use their time in the hospital as a period of vigil to make atonement for their sins and those of others. Jane was a woman who was hospitalized for weeks to receive treatment for her cancer. She told me one day that she considered her hospital room to be a place of sanctuary. It was here that she prayed for others and offered her sufferings to God. As I entered her room each day, I could not help but experience a deep peace in my soul as I felt the presence of Jesus. Although she looked to me as her physician for healing, I found in her a Good Samaritan who cared for me with her constant prayers and love. She was truly a sister in Christ to me.

Peggy was one of my patients. She had an aggressive ovarian cancer for which she received many different treatments. Despite the uncertainties she faced, she had a remarkable concern for other patients. Peggy would seek out patients who were more recently diagnosed with cancer, and she tried to spend time talking with them to provide reassurance. She also would try to give them a patient's perspective of what their treatments would be like. Peggy's quiet acts of charity touched the hearts of many other patients. This provided them with comfort and mercy.

God's mercy could permeate through many lives after one woman with advanced cancer dared to reach out to others. Such individuals are tremendous examples, particularly when we feel shy or unwilling to acknowledge another's needs or concerns.

Our Lord Jesus told St. Faustina, ... **take these graces not only for yourself, but also for others; that is, encourage the souls with whom you come in contact to trust in My infinite mercy. Oh, how I love those souls who have complete confidence in Me — I will do everything for them** (*Diary*, 294).

Beth was another patient who had multiple recurrences of a non-Hodgkin's lymphoma. Beth's disease initially seemed to be indolent. However, it transformed to a more aggressive type, and her cancer had to be treated with different therapies than would typically be used for more indolent forms of the disease. Beth's enlarged lymph nodes in her abdomen became so big that they obstructed the flow of urine from her kidneys. She needed to have stents placed by a surgeon to allow her urine to drain appropriately.

Throughout this time, Beth developed severe pain and required various medications. During her illness, the compassion of many healthcare providers moved her deeply. In addition, her husband, Tom, was a strong support. He was with her day and night, bringing her back and forth to the hospital and then caring for her at home. Over time, Beth's lymphoma responded well to treatment, and she was free of the disease years later.

As Beth overcame the disease, she was motivated to reach out to others. With her strength restored, she became a full-time caregiver for her elderly mother and a sister who was chronically ill. After experiencing the infinite mercy of God, Beth, in turn, became an instrument of mercy. She responded to Jesus' call as she helped feed the hungry, give drink to the thirsty, clothe the naked, and care for the sick. Beth's renewed life was a marvelous testimony of how God can transform the lives of those with severe illnesses, helping them bring His great mercy to the world.

Other remarkable people donate blood and bone marrow regularly for cancer patients. Though this may sometimes seem insignificant to those who donate, in fact, their gift is often a life-saving act. The donated blood or bone marrow infuses new life into patients. The donors, through their charity, help "preach" the Gospel message of mercy and love. Such merciful people can help facilitate divine healing and forgiveness to others in need.

In oncology, many souls put Jesus' words into action every day. Paula was a woman I helped care for who had an abrupt recurrence of leukemia. As I informed Paula and her husband of this, she looked at me with great love and said how hard my job must be to have to tell people such bad news. Although she was sick from her disease and may have rightfully focused on herself, the selfless concern she showed me touched my heart deeply. This increased my love for her and her family. Thus, Paula produced more fruit for the Lord's kingdom despite her seemingly weak condition in the eyes of the world.

Also of great importance is prayer for the poor souls in purgatory. Saint Faustina wrote in her *Diary* of a sister who had died appearing to her in terrible condition, all in flames with her face painfully distorted. Though initially St. Faustina's prayers and those of her religious community did not appear to help this sister who was in purgatory, later she reappeared to St. Faustina with a radiant face and her eyes beaming with joy. She told St. Faustina that she had a great love for neighbor and that many other souls profited from her prayers. She implored St. Faustina not to stop praying for the souls in purgatory (see *Diary*, 58).

Likewise, those with cancer and everyone else can unite their prayers to help the souls in purgatory. In purgatory, the work of healing continues. We must not stop praying and offering acts of mercy and love for such souls. This allows one to help in the Lord's work of healing these souls and restoring them to perfect spiritual health.

Sue was a woman whose husband, Mark, had been hospitalized in critical condition after receiving treatment for his cancer. She stood by him faithfully, sacrificing her sleep and energy to support Mark at every moment. Sue was a delightful lady. She constantly talked, and one could sit back and spend hours with her. However, sometimes it was difficult to stop her talking so the healthcare staff could focus on Mark.

She told me one day a physician told her that he did not want to speak more with her, but he wished to speak with Mark alone. This upset Sue. After all, she was an integral part of her husband's life. She had been at his side for 50 years, not to mention the many days of constant vigil spent with Mark during that hospitalization. Sue said she felt she was being pushed away.

However, even in the midst of her frustration, she let me know that as a Christian she forgave that physician. Sue removed the focus from herself to that of Jesus. I truly believe that her great faith and acts of mercy allowed her to see Christ not only in her husband, Mark, but also in the physician who offended her. As such, great healing occurred as Sue allowed the Lord's mercy to work through her life.

After Mark's death, I spoke again with Sue, and she let me know how much she missed him. Her two sons and their families provided her support, which helped her go on during her time of sorrow. As a woman of faith, she could continue on in her life of prayer, including offering up things for Mark. This opportunity enabled her to praise and thank the Lord for her beautiful marriage.

Her prayers and sacrifices could also help purify Mark of his sins on his way home to God. In particular, she could join with others to pray the Chaplet of Divine Mercy. Even though she was faithful to her wedding vows for over 50 years in fulfillment of the words, "until death do us part," Sue's devotion and love for Mark was never-ending. Thus, the loved ones of those afflicted by cancer may help bring them the Lord's healing in this life as well as in the next.

Cancer patients may find that many caring souls commonly enter into their lives. For instance, some patients say they do not know how they could have completed treatment if it were not for the compassion and support of their nurses. Often, nurses work long hours away from their families and are underpaid. Furthermore, they are exposed to great demands not only from patients and their families but also from other healthcare professionals. When some cancer patients reflect on their treatments, they see the faces of the nurses who were quietly by their sides offering words of encouragement and hope.

Physicians and other healthcare providers have been entrusted with wonderful gifts that may facilitate healing for many who are ill. They must have a deep appreciation for the knowledge and wisdom God granted them. With these talents, they have tremendous opportunities to demonstrate compassion to those in need. This great responsibility must never be neglected. To be true instruments of the Lord's mercy, healthcare workers should humbly recognize it is God working through them that results in healing. To be faithful to this call, these individuals need to be people of prayer.

Rich was an oncologist I came to know well through my career. He developed a deep prayer life early in his medical training. This helped form him into the physician he was called to be. Rich arose early each morning and consecrated everything that he would do that day to the Lord. He then would begin his day by participating in the celebration of Holy Mass. Rich told me that this was without question the most important part of his day. In the Holy Mass, the Church on earth is united with heaven as we celebrate Christ's perfect sacrifice. It is here that we are most closely united in this life with Almighty God, the Blessed Virgin Mary, and all the angels and saints.

Rich considered this time with the Lord similar to the three Apostles' experience at Jesus' Transfiguration on the mountain. Rich knew that at Mass, he also was at the top of that mountain with the Lord. There, he could obtain forgiveness for his sins each day to restore and deepen his relationship with Jesus. He reflected on God the Father's words at the Transfiguration,

"This is My beloved Son, with whom I am well pleased; listen to Him" (Mt 17:5). Rich would pay close attention to God's Word during the readings at Mass. Next, he would listen intently to the priests' homilies to help him better understand how best to apply the Holy Scriptures to his own life.

Rich also tried to further contemplate God's mercy during Mass by reflecting more on the prayers. In particular, he treasured the priest's prayer after the "Our Father" which proclaimed, "Deliver us, Lord, from every evil, and grant us peace in our day. In Your mercy keep us free from sin and protect us from all anxiety as we wait in joyful hope for the coming of our Savior, Jesus Christ." Rich then further invoked God's forgiveness with the congregation by praying, "Lamb of God, You take away the sins of the world. Have mercy on us." After encountering the Lord's glory and mercy in the Holy Eucharist, he would spend some time in Eucharistic Adoration in thanksgiving to God. Then Rich would "come down the mountain" as he left church to enter his work day.

Rich shared with me that as he drove to work each morning, he would pray the Holy Rosary or the Chaplet of The Divine Mercy for the many souls who needed his assistance. Throughout his day, he would look for brief moments here and there to pause and talk to God. He sometimes would offer up prayerful ejaculations in thanksgiving or praise to Jesus. These short periods would strengthen him to continue in his holy work.

Rich had the opportunity to care for complex cancer patients facing life-threatening diseases. His career brought him in contact with many who were afraid, alone, and dying. Some had complicated social situations, and Rich often found himself working hard with their families as well.

Despite the long hours he spent with his patients, he appreciated that these individuals gave meaning to his life. Even when Rich was not the primary physician responsible for care, he would take time to visit his patients when they were hospitalized. He listened to their concerns and offered words of encouragement. Sometimes he joked with them or shared some things from his personal life. This helped him foster many long-lasting relationships. Rich tried to see Jesus in each of his cancer patients, and he wanted to let them know he loved them.

Rich also treasured The Divine Mercy message, and this became the central focus of his vocation as a hematologist/oncologist. For those patients who were near death, he would pray the Chaplet of The Divine Mercy as a powerful means to help bring them healing. Sometimes he reminded them that none of us are God and that only God alone knows how long our lives will last in this world. Rich prayed for others to trust in God, for he knew that this is the most certain way to receive the Lord's mercy.

He thought about Jesus' words to St. Faustina, **I desire that you know more profoundly the love that burns in My Heart for souls, and you will understand this when you meditate upon My Passion. Call upon My mercy on behalf of sinners; I desire their salvation** (*Diary*, 186). This inspired Rich to continually invoke God's mercy for all souls.

To grow in his love for God and others, Rich offered up various sacrifices. Sometimes he would fast and miss meals, which allowed him to focus more clearly on spiritual matters while at work. This also allowed him to experience solidarity with the many cancer patients who could not eat. He could then have a share in their sufferings and thus better appreciate what they had to endure. On other occasions, Rich would practice moderation with many of things he enjoyed. This enabled him to experience a small portion of what his patients had to bear.

As he shared these insights with me, it was clear how showing mercy to others should be central not only to a physician's life but to everyone's. We may, then, embrace those who are suffering in love and be God's face, hands, and voice.

CHAPTER TWO

Evangelization

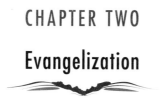

Sharing the Gospel message has always been an important ministry of the Catholic Church. Jesus instructed us, "Go, therefore, and make disciples of all nations, baptizing them in the name of the Father, and of the Son, and of the Holy Spirit, teaching them to observe all that I have commanded you. And behold, I am with you always, until the end of the age" (Mt 28:19-20).

The message of Divine Mercy is an integral part of the Gospel. This is a fundamental truth our Lord wants the world to know and believe deeply. As we experience this great gift of forgiveness, it is only natural that we would want to share it with others.

From the Old Testament, we hear how the Lord commands us to proclaim the truth to others, particularly when they have fallen from grace. He told the Prophet Ezekiel, "If a virtuous man turns away from virtue and does wrong when I place a stumbling block before him, he shall die. He shall die for his sin, and his virtuous deeds shall not be remembered; but I will hold you responsible for his death if you did not warn him. When, on the other hand, you have warned a virtuous man not to sin, and he has in fact not sinned, he shall surely live because of the warning, and you shall save your own life" (Ezek 3:20-21).

From the Gospel, Jesus teaches us how we should share His mercy. For He said, "You are the light of the world. A city set on a mountain cannot be hidden. Nor do they light a lamp and then put it under a bushel basket; it is set on a lamp stand, where it gives light to all in the house. Just so, your light must shine before others, that they may see your good deeds and glorify your heavenly Father" (Mt 5:14-16).

So, too, St. Paul said, "... we are ambassadors for Christ, as if God were appealing through us. We implore you on behalf of Christ, be reconciled to God." (2 Cor 5:20). He also tells us, "... proclaim the word; be persistent whether it is convenient or inconvenient; convince, reprimand, encourage through all patience and teaching" (2 Tim 4:2).

Jesus told St. Faustina, **Souls who spread the honor of My mercy I shield through their entire lives as a tender mother her infant, and at the hour of death I will not be a Judge for them, but the Merciful Savior** (*Diary*, 1075). We may be further inspired to evangelize by contemplating these words of the Lord to St. Faustina: **My daughter, look into My Merciful Heart and reflect its compassion in your own heart and in your deeds, so that you, who proclaim My mercy to the world, may yourself be aflame with it** (*Diary*, 1688).

Although the Gospel message is often proclaimed in word and deed to those who are ill from cancer, many such patients are already holy individuals who teach others about God. I have encountered innumerable patients who have instructed me (and others) how to live a deeper Catholic faith. They proclaim the Gospel boldly, and often their voices are soft or they "speak" through actions. Their love, appreciation, and virtuous lives give witness to the Christian way of life. These souls illustrate St. Francis of Assisi's words: "Proclaim the Gospel constantly, and, if necessary, use words."

Cancer patients often spread the Lord's kingdom through their daily acts of love. Michelle was a patient who used to tell me at each visit, "God bless you, and I will keep you in my prayers." Although this may have seemed simple to say, Michelle meant it from the bottom of her heart. Amid her great love, she encountered much suffering from the effects of her disease and from chemotherapy. Michelle tried to live each day the best she could. This was extremely difficult when she did not feel well.

Despite these challenges, she maintained her spirit of prayerfulness that she freely shared with others. Her concern for other people was remarkable, and she proclaimed the

Gospel boldly with her life of humility. Eventually, Michelle died, but her family continued her prayer life, as they were deeply affected by this woman of great love. Seeing such patients pray for their caregivers has also helped change my life. Other medical staff and I witness the Lord's infinite mercy ceaselessly radiating down upon us through these holy souls.

Some cancer patients have roommates while hospitalized. Often they come from different backgrounds and may have conflicting views on life. During their time together, though, some develop deep friendships and witness to their faith in Jesus. At times, this is all that is needed for a roommate to convert to a life in Christ. We have been told that the Lord uses some to scatter the seed, some to water and fertilize it, and others to reap the harvest for Him. When a patient with cancer is dying, his or her roommate may be the only one with the patient offering consolation and love.

Such a roommate may be likened to the good thief who died on the cross next to Jesus. This man said, "Jesus, remember me when you come into Your kingdom." Christ replied to him, "Amen, I say to you, today you will be with Me in Paradise" (Lk 23:42-43).

Father Albert is a priest I knew well during my work as a hematologist/oncologist. He instructed that although not all of us can perform heroic acts of faith and virtue like the canonized saints, we can spread the kingdom of God to those around us. Father Albert would say that if we just cooperate each day with the Lord and use the graces He gives us, we, too, can have tremendous effects on the world.

Often, it is the simple things in life that the Lord calls us to do particularly well. This allows us to proclaim the Gospel effectively wherever we find ourselves. If we consecrate all that we do to God each day, we can be certain this pleases Him. By doing the small things in life well, we may find the Lord further increasing our gifts to do greater things. For Jesus said, "Who, then, is the faithful and prudent servant, whom the master has put in charge of his household to distribute to them their food at the proper time? Blessed is that servant whom his master on his arrival finds doing so. Amen, I say to you, he will put him in charge of all his property" (Mt 24:45-47).

Many with cancer have come to realize the profound importance of living for today. This mindset has allowed numerous patients to overcome great obstacles. In particular, many cancer survivors embrace this attitude, one that is useful for everyone. None of us know when the Lord will call us from this earthly life. Consequently, we must always be vigilant and prepared for our Master's coming.

Carl was a man who was cured from a highly aggressive cancer. He was out of work for many months as he underwent cycle after cycle of intense chemotherapy in the hospital. During this time, he reflected on life, and his faith in God increased. While undergoing his treatments, Carl came to know two women, Marty and Joann, who also had the same type of cancer as he did. Occasionally, they would see each other when they returned for outpatient appointments or hospitalizations, and their friendships flourished over this time.

Although each did well initially, only Carl was cured of his cancer. He may have wondered why he survived while Marty and Joann died from the disease. They were all of similar ages and were previously healthy before their cancers were diagnosed. Yet Carl recognized his second chance at life was a gift from God.

As he recovered fully, Carl returned to work in a hospital and to his day-to-day life. However, like so many people who survive life-threatening cancers, he changed. Carl was grateful for the opportunity to serve others again and was able to proclaim the Gospel. From his healing, he could begin to live mercifully. As cancer survivors like Carl experience Divine Mercy, they can help spread this message of hope by letting others know of God's infinite love and forgiveness. Thus, they can help others make Divine Mercy a way of life. As we allow God to work in our lives, others can receive the healing they need.

In Luke's Gospel, Jesus sent 72 of His disciples ahead of Him in pairs to every town and place He intended to visit. Jesus said to them, "The harvest is abundant but the laborers are few;

so ask the master of the harvest to send out laborers for his harvest. Go on your way; behold I am sending you like lambs among wolves. Carry no money bag, no sack, no sandals; and greet no one along the way. Into whatever house you enter, first say, 'Peace to this household.' If a peaceful person lives there, your peace will rest on him; but if not, it will return to you. Stay in the same house and eat and drink what is offered to you, for the laborer deserves his payment. Do not move about from one house to another. Whatever town you enter and they welcome you, eat what is set before you, cure the sick in it and say to them, 'The kingdom of God is at hand for you'" (Lk 10:1-9).

As our Lord's servants, we must proclaim His mercy to the world. Those with cancer may actively do this as well, regardless of their condition or physical strength. Such individuals can offer their acts, words, and prayers of mercy to spread this urgent Divine Mercy message throughout a world in deep need of God's healing.

When considering how best to accomplish this work, we should reflect on Jesus' words to the 72 disciples. First, he sends them out in pairs. It is important to have support whenever one is performing work of this nature. The partner provides assistance and encouragement.

Next, one must ask God, the Harvest Master, for the aid we need to accomplish His holy work. Despite being sent out into a hostile world among wolves, Jesus tells us not to bring material support. We are to rely on God alone.

Third, Jesus tells us to focus on one place at a time. It is not necessary to travel all over the world to evangelize. By concentrating our efforts on the time and place where we find ourselves each day, we can be assured we are accomplishing what the Lord asks of us.

Linda was a woman whose husband, Ed, had multiple medical problems. They both were people of great faith. Together, their lives proclaimed the Gospel message to others. I later reflected how much they were like one of the holy pairs of disciples Jesus sent ahead of Him during his travels through Israel.

Ed's health problems included a blood cancer that progressively worsened over time. Prior to this disease, he had also been treated for bladder cancer. With the development of his blood disease, he started to have active bleeding into his urine. During this time, Ed required large numbers of blood and platelet transfusions to maintain his life. Eventually, his bladder was removed to prevent further life-threatening hemorrhages. Linda faithfully remained at Ed's side throughout this time, and she was a wonderful caregiver. It was clear that her strength came from a deep prayer life, which she continued to share with her husband.

Despite all the medications, transfusions, and other medical care Ed received, Linda's compassion for him helped him most to live each day. Her constant support during his difficult times was a great channel of the Lord's mercy. As patients like Ed encounter anxiety, fear, and suffering from their cancers, God uses others like Linda to bring about true healing through mercy.

After Ed's death, Linda's love for him did not cease, as she continued to pray for him. Shortly after, she became a volunteer at the hospital. Linda told me she had witnessed tremendous compassion from those who helped care for Ed, and she knew that she now had to share this with others. As a woman of great faith, Linda sought ways to be merciful to others suffering from various illnesses. She visited one patient at a time, not worrying what she was to say, for she knew the Lord would give her the words she needed. We are all part of the Lord's family, and just as our heavenly Father is merciful, so, too, each of His children must be. Living with compassion for others manifests Christ's presence to all in need throughout the world.

During our lives and particularly during prayer, it is sometimes necessary to detach from the world. As we contemplate the greatness of our Lord and His infinite mercy, we are left in awe. We then pray to place others in our Lord's hands. We pray for their full union with Him. Everything we have comes from God. They are His possessions. However, due to the free will that God gives each of us, we have the ability to either accept or reject Him and His mercy. Man and woman are the only part of God's creation that may be lost by sin. Therefore, we have a great obligation to pray for others and to help evangelize so no one will be lost.

Physicians, nurses, and other healthcare providers have unique opportunities to care for those afflicted with cancer and other illnesses. Administration of medical therapies may be of great value, as it offers patients the possibility of physical healing. However, far more important is assisting in spiritual healing. The body and soul are intimately related. If either one is ailing, it affects the other. Many healthcare providers are people of faith who can share this great gift with those in need. In doing so, patients may experience The Divine Mercy message and receive God's healing power.

Debbie was a delightful woman, not a Christian. She developed a blood cancer that had been successfully treated, and she remained well for more than a year. However, later the cancer relapsed in her central nervous system. Debbie's condition rapidly worsened, and she became weaker. She could no longer walk and then lost all of the strength in her legs. I sensed she was becoming depressed despite taking her antidepressant medication. Debbie's family was extremely supportive, particularly when she was dying.

The last time I saw her, she told me how horrible my job must be. She asked how I could possibly do the work I do each day. She could not fathom how I could repeatedly tell people that their deaths were imminent. As I thought about her question, many things came to my mind. Speaking about death is difficult with anyone. However, I find it particularly challenging to do it with patients like Debbie, whom I have known well over a long period of time. Yet rather than fearing or avoiding such discussions, I have found them to be opportunities in which I can share the Lord's grace with others.

As Debbie and I spoke further, she seemed more frustrated. She knew that she was unable to complete many of the things she desired to accomplish in life. I prayed the Chaplet of The Divine Mercy for her and sought the best way that I could bring Jesus Christ and The Divine Mercy message into her life. It then occurred to me that as part of the Body of

Christ, I was able to bring Jesus directly to Debbie at that instant. We are all called to bear Jesus to the world, since He lives within each member of His Body. By showing her compassion, support, and love, I had a tremendous opportunity to bring Jesus into Debbie's life.

I told her how blessed she was to have a family that she loved and who loved her, for love is what makes us a success in this life as well as in the next, not material possessions, worldly power, or a long life. Debbie seemed encouraged by this, and I felt that she experienced the Lord's mercy and healing.

After her death, I spoke to her sister, who seemed to think that Debbie failed as she died from her cancer. I tried to console her and reassure her that Debbie's life was a success. Regardless of whether we die from cancer, a heart attack, a motor vehicle accident, or anything else, it is clear our mortal lives in this world are transient. Therefore, one form of death is not ultimately worse than another. The end is the same, with a transition from our earthly existence to our next life for eternity. The only matter of importance is whether one's eternity is with or without God. Those who seek the Lord and confidently trust in His mercy in this life will allow God to welcome them home into His kingdom forever.

At the hospital where I work, translators assist patients who do not speak English to communicate with their healthcare providers. The more complex a patient's medical condition, the more time and effort the translator must spend to help bring about a clear understanding between patient and physician.

Sheila was a patient who spoke a different language than me. She required a bone marrow transplant for her advanced blood disease. It took hours for us to communicate through a translator for her to have a good understanding of the procedure. This included a thorough explanation of the risks, the potential benefits that could be obtained, the alternatives if she chose not to pursue the treatment, and the personnel who would be involved in her care. These things had to be explained in detail to Sheila, so she could give informed consent for the treatment.

In a similar manner, we are all called to be effective translators for the Lord to bring his Gospel message to the world. Just as priests and religious carry out their work for the Church, we, the lay faithful, are also called to bring the transforming power of the Gospel to the world. By taking time to share our Lord's Word, we can reach many souls who are in deep need of God's mercy. Regardless of the time needed to accomplish the task, we must be clear to others about the spiritual risks of following Christ.

These include suffering, misunderstanding, rejection, and persecution by others. For Jesus told us, "If the world hates you, realize that it hated Me first. ... 'No slave is greater than his master.' If they persecuted Me, they will also persecute you" (Jn 15:18, 20). A far worse risk that we must inform others about is falling away from the faith, including the real possibility of hell for those who still reject our merciful God.

The benefits of accepting Jesus as our Lord and Savior are true peace and life on high with Almighty God in His kingdom for all eternity. The spiritual alternative is rejection of God and hell. The personnel involved in God's work are all the faithful who follow His Word. Thus, it is critical to present these spiritual matters clearly to others in order for them to be informed, so they may freely consent to accept God's mercy.

In the Gospel, we read how Jesus expelled a demon from a mute person, and the crowds were amazed. The Pharisees then criticized Jesus, saying He drove out demons by the prince of demons (see Mt 12:22-24). Many today need the Lord to heal them from a mute spirit that prohibits them from spreading the Gospel message. Often these are good people, but they are astonishingly reserved when it comes to speaking about their faith. In some instances, certain souls are not well formed in the faith, and naturally it is difficult for them to share it with others. The Lord's grace and gift of faith are readily available to all who ask, seek, and knock at the door (see Mt 7:7-8).

Others may be well formed in the faith, and some may be gifted speakers who are well versed, yet fear keeps them

250 | Divine Mercy, Triumph over Cancer

mute. By coming to know our Lord's mercy and infinite goodness, one's fear disappears. Then they may become useful servants for the Lord. Just as some Pharisees tried to criticize Jesus for expelling the demon from the person who was mute, others try to silence those freed from sin who speak of God's great mercy. This great message of hope refreshes our hearts and all who will listen in this broken world.

As I reflect on many of my prior teachers and mentors, I recall the vast number of cancer patients that I have had the privilege to know and care for over the years. I often feel like a student listening to his teacher as I sit at their bedsides.

In many cases, patients may be considerably younger than me or with far less "formal" education. However, during Jesus' public life of teaching, He, too, was considerably younger than other teachers. It was presumed that He had no formal education in the eyes of the religious leaders of His time. Nonetheless, He was God, the Word who became flesh and dwelt among us. The Lord may speak through anyone.

From interacting with cancer patients, I have had the opportunity to learn more from them than volumes of textbooks could teach. Christ's life is present, and His work continues in all such souls. This is confirmed by the concluding words of St. John's Gospel, "There are also many other things that Jesus did, but if these were to be described individually, I do not think the whole world would contain the books that would be written" (Jn 21:25).

Many cancer patients are blessed in this life with others who have loved them. However, everyone should be comforted to know that we are all certainly loved by our God. In turn, many patients love others deeply as they live and die with their cancers. No matter what their past may have been, such individuals can pour out the love they have received from Almighty God and others.

We can only give what we have received. Therefore, the gift of love and mercy from our Divine Savior Jesus Christ is to be given to all. Saint Faustina had a clear understanding of this as she said, "I see now that my deeds which have flowed from love are more perfect than those which I have done out of fear. I have placed my trust in God and fear nothing. I have given myself over to His holy will; let Him do with me as He wishes, and I will still love Him" (*Diary*, 589).

Those with cancer often bear incredible suffering that can be a source of sanctity for them and the world if they offer it up for the glory of God. For in saying "not my will but Your will be done" to Almighty God, they become like Jesus and allow His redemptive suffering to be applied through their lives.

Healthcare providers and researchers have made considerable progress in our understanding of cancer and in ways to treat such disease, but there is more to learn. Those working in this discipline understand that the more we know, the more we realize how much we do not yet know.

Likewise, in our spiritual lives, the closer we grow in our relationships with Almighty God, the more we come to realize how limited our understanding is of His unfathomable mercy, goodness, and love. After St. Peter and his companions had been fishing unsuccessfully all night, Jesus told him to go out into deep water and lower his nets (see Lk 5:1-11). Saint Peter trusted the Lord and caught an incredible amount of fish. Their boats were at the point of sinking from the enormous catch. The Lord also calls each of us to go deeper, that we may grow in our love and trust of Him.

Jesus told St. Faustina, **When a soul approaches Me with trust, I fill it with such an abundance of graces that it cannot contain them within itself, but radiates them to other souls** (*Diary*, 1074). St. Faustina also prayed, "O Holy Trinity, Eternal God, I want to shine in the crown of Your mercy as a tiny gem whose beauty depends on the ray of Your light and of Your inscrutable mercy" (*Diary*, 617).

Countless patients with cancer have radiated such grace to the world around them. I have been blessed beyond measure to have had the opportunity daily to walk among these individuals, many of whom are the saints our world may never know. The faith of such souls and their trust in Divine Mercy enables them to triumph over cancer. In union with that of the holy Catholic

Church, my hope and prayer is that The Divine Mercy will continue to permeate and transform all lives until we are all one with God in His kingdom for all eternity. Therefore, with St. Faustina and all the saints, we should continually proclaim, "Jesus, I trust in You!"

Glossary of Selected Medical Terms

Aplastic anemia – a medical condition that is characterized by an empty bone marrow resulting in extremely low blood counts, which predispose patients to life-threatening bleeding and infections

Biologic therapy – a cancer treatment that affects tumors predominantly through the action of natural host defense mechanisms or the administration of natural substances from mammals

Cancer – a disease that is characterized by the development of abnormal cells in part of a person's body that accumulate and then may invade and destroy surrounding tissues. Over time, these abnormal cells may spread to more distant parts of the body where they may have further destructive effects

Chronic myeloproliferative disorder – a group of medical conditions that are characterized by overproduction of certain types of blood cells from the bone marrow; over time, patients may develop progressive bone marrow failure or transformation of the disease to acute leukemia

Graft-vs.-host disease – a condition that may develop in some patients after receiving a blood or bone marrow transplant that results from the new blood cells derived from the donor (the graft) attacking parts of the patient's body (the host); although this disease may affect many different organs, the skin, intestines and liver are the most commonly involved

Hand-foot syndrome – a side effect that may occur after certain chemotherapy treatments in which the hands and feet of patients may become red and painful with some individuals experiencing peeling of the skin

Hematology (hematologic) – the study of blood and its disorders

Leukemia – a group of blood cancers characterized by an overproduction of abnormal white blood cells. This results in extremely low normal blood counts that predispose patients to life-threatening bleeding and infections; some types may result in enlargement of the lymph nodes, spleen, and liver; some forms are aggressive and grow rapidly (acute), while others may have more indolent disease courses (chronic)

Lymphoma – a group of cancers involving the lymphatic system; these diseases may result in progressive, increasing size of the lymph nodes, spleen, and liver; these cancers may also involve the bone marrow and over time result in low blood counts that predispose patients to life-threatening bleeding and infections

Malignancy (malignant) – a cancer

Multiple myeloma – a blood cancer that results from an accumulation of abnormal plasma cells in the bone marrow; this may result in progressive bone marrow failure that predisposes patients to life-threatening bleeding and infections; the disease may also result in kidney failure, or it may affect the bones including the development of fractures

Myelodysplastic syndrome (myelodysplasia) – a group of blood conditions characterized by a defect in the maturation of bone marrow cells that result in extremely low blood counts, which predispose patients to life-threatening bleeding and infections; over time, this condition transforms to acute leukemia

Neuropathy – a disease that affects the peripheral nerves and that may cause weakness, numbness, or pain in the affected body part

Oncology – the study of cancer

Pathogens – a microorganism, such as a bacterium, virus, or fungus, which parasitizes a human, animal, or plant and produces a disease

Toxicity – the degree to which a substance or treatment is poisonous

Tracheostomy – a surgical procedure in which a hole is made through the neck into the trachea (windpipe) to relieve obstruction to breathing; a curved tube is usually inserted through the hole

Selected Bibliography

Barrette, G. *Spiritual direction in the Roman Catholic tradition.* Journal of Psychology and Theology Vol. 30(4), 2002.

Came, David. *Pope Benedict's Divine Mercy Mandate.* Stockbridge, Mass.: Marian Press, 2009.

Flynn, Vinny. *7 Secrets of the Eucharist.* Stockbridge, Mass.: MercySong, 2006.

John Paul II. Encyclical Letter *Rich in Mercy (Dives in Misericordia)*, 1980.

John Paul II. Apostolic Letter *Salvific Suffering (Salvifici Doloris)*, February 11, 1984.

Kowalska, Saint Maria Faustina. *Diary of Saint Maria Faustina Kowalska: Divine Mercy in My Soul.* Stockbridge, Mass.: Marian Press, 1987.

Mother Teresa. *Loving Jesus.* Cincinnati, Ohio: St. Anthony Messenger Press, 1991.

Stackpole, Robert. *Divine Mercy: a Guide from Genesis to Benedict XVI.* Stockbridge, Mass: Marian Press, 2008.

Our Lady of Fatima's "Peace Plan from Heaven." Monrovia, Calif.: Catholic Treasures, 1950.

Selected Prayers

The Holy Rosary

1.) Make the Sign of the Cross.

2.) Pray the Apostles' Creed.*

I believe in God, the Father almighty, Creator of heaven and earth, and in Jesus Christ, his only Son, our Lord, who was conceived by the Holy Spirit, born of the Virgin Mary, suffered under Pontius Pilate, was crucified, died, and was buried; he descended into hell; on the third day he rose again from the dead; he ascended into heaven, and is seated at the right hand of God the Father almighty; from there he will come to judge the living and the dead. I believe in the Holy Spirit, the holy catholic Church, the communion of saints, the forgiveness of sins, the resurrection of the body, and life everlasting. Amen.

3.) Pray the "Our Father."

Our Father, who art in heaven, hallowed be Thy name; Thy kingdom come; Thy will be done on earth as it is in heaven. Give us this day our daily bread; and forgive us our trespasses as we forgive those who trespass against us; and lead us not into temptation, but deliver us from evil. Amen.

4.) Pray three "Hail Marys."

Hail Mary, full of grace. The Lord is with thee. Blessed art thou among women, and blessed is the fruit of thy womb, Jesus. Holy Mary, Mother of God, pray for us sinners, now and at the hour of our death. Amen

---

*The wording of the Apostles' Creed conforms with the *Roman Missal*.

5.) Pray the "Glory be to the Father."
Glory be to the Father, and to the Son, and to the Holy Spirit. As it was in the beginning, is now, and ever shall be, world without end. Amen.

6.) Announce the Mystery of the Rosary to be contemplated.

a. The Joyful Mysteries
   i. The Annunciation
   ii. The Visitation
   iii. The Birth of Jesus
   iv. The Presentation of Jesus in the Temple
   v. The Finding of the Child Jesus in the Temple

b. The Luminous Mysteries
   i. The Baptism of Jesus
   ii. The Wedding at Cana
   iii. Jesus' Proclamation of the Kingdom of God
   iv. The Transfiguration of Jesus
   v. The Institution of the Most Holy Eucharist

c. The Sorrowful Mysteries
   i. The Agony in the Garden
   ii. The Scourging at the Pillar
   iii. The Crowning with Thorns
   iv. The Carrying of the Cross
   v. The Crucifixion and Death of Jesus

d. The Glorious Mysteries
   i. The Resurrection
   ii. The Ascension
   iii. The Descent of the Holy Spirit
   iv. The Assumption
   v. The Coronation of Mary Queen of Heaven and Earth

7.) Pray one "Our Father."

8.) Pray 10 "Hail Marys," while meditating on the Mystery.

9.) Pray the "Glory be to the Father."

10.) After each decade pray the following prayer requested by the Blessed Virgin Mary at Fatima:

O my Jesus, forgive us our sins, save us from the fires of hell, lead all souls to heaven, especially those in most need of Thy mercy.

11.) Announce the Second Mystery of the Rosary to be contemplated and repeat the prayers in steps 7 through 10 and then continue with the Third, Fourth and Fifth Mysteries in the same manner.

12.) Pray the "Hail, Holy Queen."

Hail, Holy Queen, Mother of Mercy, our life, our sweetness and our hope, to thee do we cry, poor banished children of Eve; to thee do we send up our sighs, mourning and weeping in this vale of tears; turn, then, most gracious Advocate, thine eyes of mercy toward us, and after this, our exile, show unto us the blessed fruit of thy womb, Jesus. O clement, O loving, O sweet Virgin Mary!

Pray for us, O holy Mother of God, that we may be made worthy of the promises of Christ.

Let us pray. O God, whose only begotten Son, by His life, death and Resurrection has purchased for us the rewards of eternal life, grant we beseech Thee that meditating upon these Mysteries of the Most Holy Rosary of the Blessed Virgin Mary, that we may imitate what they contain and obtain what they promise, through the same Christ our Lord. Amen.

13.) Pray one "Our Father," one "Hail Mary," and one "Glory be to the Father" for the intentions of our Holy Father.

14.) In general, The Joyful Mysteries are prayed on Mondays, Saturdays, and during Advent on Sundays. The Luminous Mysteries are prayed on Thursdays. The Sorrowful Mysteries are prayed on Tuesdays, Fridays, and during Lent on Sundays. The Glorious Mysteries are prayed on Wednesdays and Sundays.

The Chaplet of The Divine Mercy
(Use a rosary)

1.) Make the Sign of the Cross.

2.) Pray the optional Opening Prayer:

You expired Jesus, but the source of life gushed forth for souls, and the ocean of mercy opened up for the whole world. O Fount of Life, unfathomable Divine Mercy, envelop the whole world and empty Yourself out upon us (*Diary*, 1319).

(3 times)

O Blood and Water which gushed forth from the Heart of Jesus as a fount of mercy for us, I trust in You (*Diary*, 84).

3.) Pray the "Our Father."

Our Father, who art in heaven, hallowed be Thy name; Thy kingdom come; Thy will be done on earth as it is in heaven. Give us this day our daily bread; and forgive us our trespasses as we forgive those who trespass against us; and lead us not into temptation, but deliver us from evil. Amen.

4.) Pray the "Hail Mary."

Hail Mary, full of grace. The Lord is with thee. Blessed art thou among women, and blessed is the fruit of thy womb, Jesus. Holy Mary, Mother of God, pray for us sinners, now and at the hour of our death. Amen

5.) Pray the Apostles' Creed.

I believe in God, the Father almighty, creator of heaven and earth. I believe in Jesus Christ, His only Son, our Lord. He was conceived by the power of the Holy Spirit, and born of the Virgin Mary. He suffered under Pontius Pilate, was crucified, died, and was buried. He descended to the dead. On the third day He rose again. He ascended into heaven, and is seated at the right hand of the Father. He will come again to judge the living and the dead. I believe in the Holy Spirit, the holy Catholic Church, the communion of saints, the forgiveness of sins, the resurrection of the body, and the life everlasting. Amen.

6.) On the "Our Father" bead before each decade pray:
Eternal Father, I offer You the Body and Blood, Soul and Divinity of Your dearly beloved Son, Our Lord Jesus Christ, in atonement for our sins and those of the whole world.

7.) On the 10 "Hail Mary" beads of each of the 5 decades pray:
For the sake of His sorrowful Passion, have mercy on us and on the whole world.

8.) Pray the concluding Doxology (3 times):
Holy God, Holy Mighty One, Holy Immortal Once, have mercy on us and on the whole world.

9.) Pray the optional Concluding Prayer:
Eternal God, in whom mercy is endless and the treasury of compassion inexhaustible, look kindly upon us and increase Your mercy in us, that in difficult moments we might not despair nor become despondent, but with great confidence submit ourselves to Your holy will, which is Love and Mercy itself (*Diary*, 950).

The Praises of the Divine Mercy
(*Diary*, 948-949)
The Love of God is the flower – Mercy the fruit.

Let the doubting soul read these considerations on Divine Mercy and become trusting.

Divine Mercy, gushing forth from the bosom of the Father,
  I trust in You.
Divine Mercy, greatest attribute of God, I trust in You.
Divine Mercy, incomprehensible mystery, I trust in You.
Divine Mercy, fount gushing forth from the mystery of the Most Blessed Trinity, I trust in You.
Divine Mercy, unfathomed by any intellect, human or angelic,
  I trust in You.
Divine Mercy, from which wells forth all life and happiness,
  I trust in You.
Divine Mercy, better than the heavens, I trust in You.
Divine Mercy, source of miracles and wonders, I trust in You.

Divine Mercy, encompassing the whole universe, I trust in You.

Divine Mercy, descending to the earth in the Person of the
Incarnate Word, I trust in You.

Divine Mercy, which flowed out from the open wound of the
Heart of Jesus, I trust in You.

Divine Mercy, enclosed in the Heart of Jesus for us, and
especially for sinners, I trust in You.

Divine Mercy, unfathomed in the institution of the Sacred
Host, I trust in You.

Divine Mercy, in the founding of Holy Church, I trust in You.

Divine Mercy, in the Sacrament of Holy Baptism, I trust in You.

Divine Mercy, in our justification through Jesus Christ,
I trust in You.

Divine Mercy, accompanying us through our whole life,
I trust in You.

Divine Mercy, embracing us especially at the hour of death,
I trust in You.

Divine Mercy, endowing us with immortal life, I trust in You.

Divine Mercy, accompanying us every moment of our life,
I trust in You.

Divine Mercy, shielding us from the fire of hell, I trust in You.

Divine Mercy, in the conversion of hardened sinners,
I trust in You.

Divine Mercy, astonishment for Angels, incomprehensible to
Saints, I trust in You.

Divine Mercy, unfathomed in all the mysteries of God,
I trust in You.

Divine Mercy, lifting us out of every misery, I trust in You.

Divine Mercy, source of our happiness and joy, I trust in You.

Divine Mercy, in calling us forth from nothingness to existence,
I trust in You.

Divine Mercy, embracing all the works of His hands,
I trust in You.

Divine Mercy, crown of all of God's handiwork, I trust in You.

Divine Mercy, in which we are all immersed, I trust in You.

Divine Mercy, sweet relief for anguished hearts, I trust in You.

Divine Mercy, only hope of despairing souls, I trust in You.

Divine Mercy, repose of hearts, peace amidst fear, I trust in You.

Divine Mercy, delight and ecstasy of holy souls, I trust in You.

Divine Mercy, inspiring hope against all hope, I trust in You.

For the Grace to be Merciful to Others
(*Diary*, 948-949)

O Most Holy Trinity! As many times as I breathe, as many times as my heart beats, as many times as my blood pulsates through my body, so many thousand times do I want to glorify Your mercy.

I want to be completely transformed into Your mercy and to be Your living reflection, O Lord. May the greatest of all divine attributes, that of Your unfathomable mercy, pass through my heart and soul to my neighbor.

Help me, O Lord, that my eyes may be merciful, so that I may never suspect or judge from appearances, but look for what is beautiful in my neighbors' souls and come to their rescue.

Help me, that my ears may be merciful, so that I may give heed to my neighbors' needs and not be indifferent to their pains and moanings.

Help me, O Lord, that my tongue may be merciful, so that I should never speak negatively of my neighbor, but have a word of comfort and forgiveness for all.

Help me, O Lord, that my hands may be merciful and filled with good deeds, so that I may do only good to my neighbors and take upon myself the more difficult and toilsome tasks.

Help me, that my feet may be merciful, so that I may hurry to assist my neighbor, overcoming my own fatigue and weariness. My true rest is in the service of my neighbor.

Help me, O Lord, that my heart may be merciful so that I myself may feel all the sufferings of my neighbor. I will refuse my heart to no one. I will be sincere even with those who, I know, will abuse my kindness. And I will lock myself up in the most merciful Heart of Jesus. I will bear my own suffering in silence. May Your mercy, O Lord, rest upon me.

You Yourself command me to exercise the three degrees of mercy. The first: the act of mercy, of whatever kind. The second: the word of mercy — if I cannot carry out a work of mercy, I will assist by my words. The third: prayer — if I cannot show mercy by deeds or words, I can always do so by prayer. My prayer reaches out even there where I cannot reach out physically.

O my Jesus, transform me into Yourself, for You can do all things.

Prayer for a Merciful Heart

O Jesus, I understand that Your mercy is beyond all imagining, and therefore I ask You to make my heart so big that there will be room in it for the needs of all the souls living on the face of the earth ... and the souls suffering in Purgatory. ... Make my heart sensitive to all the sufferings of my neighbor, whether of body or soul. O my Jesus, I know that You act toward us as we act toward our neighbor. ... Make my heart like unto Your merciful Heart (*Diary*, 692) ... Transform it into Your own Heart that I may sense the needs of other hearts, especially those who are sad and suffering. May the rays of mercy rest in my heart (*Diary*, 514). ... Jesus, help me to go through life doing good to everyone (*Diary*, 692).

At the Feet of Christ in the Eucharist

O Jesus, Divine Prisoner of Love, when I consider Your love and how You emptied Yourself for me, my senses fail me. You hide your inconceivable majesty and lower Yourself to miserable me. O King of Glory, though You hide Your beauty, yet the eye of my soul rends the veil. I see the angelic choirs giving You honor without cease, and all the heavenly Powers praising You without cease, and without cease they are saying: Holy, Holy, Holy.

Oh, who will comprehend Your love and Your unfathomable mercy toward us! O Prisoner of Love, I lock up my poor heart in the tabernacle, that it may adore You without cease night and day. I know of no obstacle in this adoration, and even though I be physically distant, my heart is always with You. Nothing can put a stop to my love for You. No obstacles exist for me (*Diary*, 80).

O Holy Trinity, One and Indivisible God, may You be blessed for this great gift and testament of mercy (*Diary*, 81).

I adore You, Lord and Creator, hidden in the Blessed Sacrament. I adore You for all the works of Your hands, that reveal to me so much wisdom, goodness and mercy, O Lord. You have spread so much beauty over the earth, and it tells me about Your beauty, even though these beautiful things are but a faint reflection of You, Incomprehensible Beauty. And although You have hidden Yourself and concealed Your beauty, my eye, enlightened by faith, reaches You, and my soul recognizes its Creator, its Highest Good; and my heart is completely immersed in prayer of adoration (*Diary*, 1692).

My Lord and Creator, Your goodness encourages me to converse with You. Your mercy abolishes the chasm which separates the Creator from the creature. To converse with You, O Lord, is the delight of my heart. In You I find everything that my heart could desire. Here Your light illumines my mind, enabling it to know You more and more deeply. Here streams of graces flow down upon my heart. Here my soul draws eternal life. O my Lord and Creator, You alone, beyond all these gifts, give Your own Self to me and unite Yourself intimately with Your miserable creature (*Diary*, 1692).

O Christ, I am most delighted when I see that You are loved, and that Your praise and glory resound, especially the praise of Your mercy. O Christ, to the last moment of my life, I will not stop glorifying Your goodness and mercy. With every drop of my blood, with every beat of my heart, I glorify Your mercy. I long to be entirely transformed into a hymn of Your glory. When I find myself on my deathbed, may the last beat of my heart be a loving hymn in praise of Your unfathomable mercy (*Diary*, 1708).

Prayer for Divine Mercy

O Greatly Merciful God, Infinite Goodness, today all mankind calls out from the abyss of its misery to Your mercy — to Your compassion, O God; and it is with its mighty voice of misery that it cries out. Gracious God, do not reject the prayer of this earth's exiles! O Lord, Goodness beyond our understanding, Who are acquainted with our misery through and through, and know that by our own power we cannot ascend to You, we implore You: anticipate us with Your grace and keep on increasing Your mercy in us, that we may faithfully do Your holy will all through our life and at death's hour. Let the omnipotence of Your mercy shield us from the darts of our salvation's enemies, that we may with confidence, as Your children, await Your final coming — that day known to You alone. And we expect to obtain everything promised us by Jesus in spite of all our wretchedness. For Jesus is our Hope: Through His merciful Heart, as through an open gate, we pass through to heaven (*Diary*, 1570).

Memorare to St. Joseph

(Begin with an Our Father, Hail Mary, and Glory Be to the Father)

Remember, O most pure spouse of Mary, and my dearly beloved guardian, St. Joseph, that never was it known that anyone who invoked your care and requested your help was left without consolation.

Inspired with this confidence, I come to you, and with all the ardor of my spirit I commend myself to you. Do not reject my prayer, O Foster Father of the Savior, but graciously receive and answer it. Amen.

St. Peregrine
Patron Saint for those with Cancer

Saint Peregrine was born in 1260 at Forlì, Italy, to an affluent family. He lived a comfortable life as a youth, and politically opposed the papacy. After he experienced the forgiveness of St. Philip Benizi, he changed his life and joined the Servite Order. He was ordained a priest, and later returned to his home to establish a Servite community. There he was widely known for his preaching, penances, and counsel in the confessional. He was cured of cancer, after he received a vision of Christ on the cross reaching out His hand to touch his impaired limb. He died in 1345 and was canonized in 1726. (EWTN Global Catholic Network)

Prayer to St. Peregrine

O great and glorious wonder-worker, St. Peregrine, you have obtained numerous miracles from God for those suffering from serious illness. For so many years you suffered with cancer, and were favored by the vision of Jesus coming down from His cross to cure your affliction. We ask you to intercede on our behalf for the healing of those whom we entrust to you.

(Pause and silently recall the names of the sick for whom you are praying.)

Obtain for us, St. Peregrine, the grace to patiently endure all sufferings, so that we may, in imitation of your virtue, more profoundly love our crucified Lord, His sorrowful Mother, and through your intercession, merit glory everlasting. Amen.

Novena to St. Peregrine

Glorious wonder-worker, St. Peregrine, you answered the divine call with a ready spirit, and forsook all the comforts of a life of ease and all the empty honors of the world to dedicate yourself to God in the Order of His holy Mother.

You labored manfully for the salvation of souls. In union with Jesus crucified, you endured painful sufferings with such patience as to deserve to be healed miraculously of an incurable cancer in your leg by a touch of His divine hand.

Obtain for me the grace to answer every call of God and to fulfill His will in all the events of life. Enkindle in my heart a consuming zeal for the salvation of all men.

Deliver me from the infirmities that afflict my body (*especially...*).

Obtain for me also a perfect resignation to the sufferings it may please God to send me, so that, imitating our crucified Savior and His sorrowful Mother, I may merit eternal glory in heaven.

St. Peregrine, pray for me and for all who invoke your aid.

Caring for the Poor

Ten percent of the proceeds from sales of *Divine Mercy, Triumph over Cancer* will be donated to the medical outreach of Eucharistic Apostles of The Divine Mercy (EADM), an apostolate of the Marian Fathers of the Immaculate Conception.

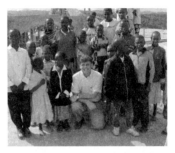

EADM's medical outreach involves shipping cargo containers of mostly medical supplies, along with clothing and religious items, to the poor and marginalized in developing countries. Currently, the apostolate has shipped more

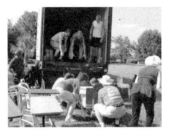

than 125 containers with donated items valued at more than $25 million. Containers have been sent to Ghana, Nigeria, Tanzania, Uganda, Cameroon, Rwanda, Ukraine, Mexico, the Dominican Republic, Ecuador, Peru, Honduras, Nicaragua, India, the Philippines, and Cuba.

The apostolate also plans to open a small medical and dental clinic in a poor region on the island of Mindanao in the Philippines. The clinic, which will be near a large Divine Mercy Shrine in El Salvador on

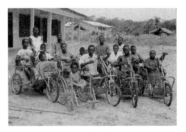

Mindanao, will serve the local people with care and dignity. In planning for the clinic, EADM's Director Bryan Thatcher, MD, is working closely with the Marian Fathers, who have missionaries serving in the Philippines.

For more information on EADM, please call 1-877-380-0727 or visit www.thedivinemercy.org/eadm

Join the
Association of Marian Helpers,
headquartered at the
National Shrine of The Divine Mercy,
and share in special blessings!

**An invitation from
Fr. Joseph, MIC, the director**

Marian Helpers is an Association of Christian faithful of the Congregation of Marian Fathers of the Immaculate Conception. By becoming a member, you share in the spiritual benefits of the daily Masses, prayers, and good works of the Marian priests and brothers. This is a special offer of grace given to you by the Church through the Marian Fathers. Please consider this opportunity to share in these blessings, along with others whom you would wish to join into this spiritual communion.

Enroll Loved Ones!

Give a Consoling Gift: *Prayer*

Enroll your loved ones in the Association of Marian Helpers. Enrollments can be offered for the living or deceased. We offer a variety of enrollment cards: wedding, anniversary, First Holy Communion, birthday, get well, and more.

Request a Mass
to be offered by the Marian Fathers
for your loved one:
Individual Masses
(for the living or deceased)
Gregorian Masses
(30 days of consecutive Masses for the deceased)

1-800-462-7426
Marian.org/Enrollments   **Marian.org/Mass**

ESSENTIAL DIVINE MERCY RESOURCES

DIARY OF SAINT MARIA FAUSTINA KOWALSKA: DIVINE MERCY IN MY SOUL

The *Diary* chronicles the message that Jesus, the Divine Mercy, gave to the world through this humble nun. In it, we are reminded to trust in His forgiveness — and as Christ is merciful, so, too, are we instructed to be merciful to others. Written in the 1930s, this message exemplifies God's love toward mankind and, to this day, remains a source of hope and renewal. Keep the *Diary* next to your Bible for constant insight and inspiration for your spiritual growth!

LARGE PAPERBACK: Y65-NBFD
COMPACT PAPERBACK: Y65-DNBF
DELUXE LEATHER-BOUND EDITION: Y65-DDBURG
AUDIO DIARY MP3 EDITION: Y65-ADMP3
*e*book: Y65-EDIARY

THE DIVINE MERCY MESSAGE AND DEVOTION

Fr. Seraphim Michalenko, MIC, with Vinny Flynn and Robert A. Stackpole

Includes all elements and essential prayers of the Divine Mercy message and devotion.
Y65-M17 *e*book: Y65-EBM17

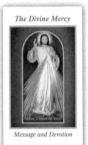

The Divine Mercy

Jesus, I Trust in You!

Message and Devotion

DIVINE MERCY 101 KIT

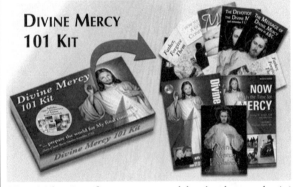

Includes: *The Divine Mercy Explained* booklet, *Now is the Time for Mercy* book, *Divine Mercy 101* DVD, prayercards, and pamphlets on works of mercy, Confession, forgiveness, and more.
Y65-DMKIT

Now is the time for mercy — and here's where to begin! Compact, practical, this kit offers the basics of the Divine Mercy message and devotion, helping you answer God's call to receive His mercy and share that mercy with the world.

Call 1-800-462-7426 or visit ShopMercy.org

Essential Divine Mercy Resources

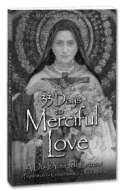

33 Days to Merciful Love
A Do-It-Yourself Retreat in Preparation for Consecration to Divine Mercy

Live Divine Mercy to the full! Get your copy of *33 Days to Merciful Love* by Fr. Michael Gaitley, MIC, the stirring sequel to the international sensation, *33 Days to Morning Glory*. Using the same 33-day preparation format, *33 Days to Merciful Love* journeys with one of the most beloved saints of modern times, St. Thérèse of Lisieux, and concludes with a consecration to Divine Mercy. So whether you want to deepen your love of Divine Mercy or have a devotion to St. Thérèse, *33 Days to Merciful Love* is the book for you. Paperback, 216 pages.

Y65-33DML   *e*book: Y65-EB33DML

THE SECOND GREATEST STORY EVER TOLD
Fr. Michael E. Gaitley, MIC

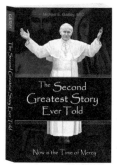

In *The Second Greatest Story Ever Told,* bestselling author Fr. Michael Gaitley, MIC, reveals St. John Paul II's witness for our time. Building on the prophetic voices of Sts. Margaret Mary Alacoque, Thérèse of Lisieux, Maximilian Kolbe, and Faustina Kowalska, *The Second Greatest Story Ever Told* is more than a historical account of the Great Mercy Pope. This book expounds on the profound connection between Divine Mercy and Marian consecration. It serves as an inspiration for all those who desire to bear witness to the mercy of God, focused on Christ and formed by Mary. Now is the time of mercy. Now is the time to make John Paul's story your own. Paperback, 240 pages.

Y65-SGSBK
*e*book: Y65-EBSGSBK

DIVINE MERCY IN THE SECOND GREATEST STORY (DVD AND GUIDEBOOK)

Exciting 10-part series with DVD and workbook hosted and written by Fr. Michael Gaitley and based on his best-selling book *The Second Greatest Story Ever Told.*

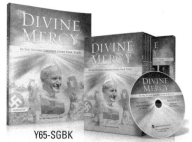

Y65-SGBK

Y65-SGDVD

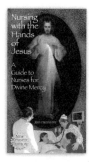

For Doctors and Nurses:
NURSING WITH THE HANDS OF JESUS
A GUIDE TO NURSES FOR DIVINE MERCY

by Marie Romagnano, RN

The first spiritual guide on the Divine Mercy message and devotion specifically for nurses and those who care for the sick, injured, and dying. A practical "how-to" guide. 88 pages, pocket-size. Y65-NTHJ

Call 1-800-462-7426 or visit ShopMercy.org

ESSENTIAL DIVINE MERCY RESOURCES

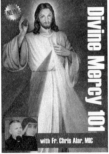
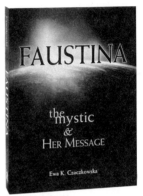
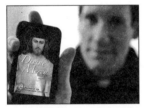